Powerful Ketogenic Diet and Intermittent Fasting Secrets

Complete Keto Fast Guide to Gain the Low-Carb Clarity Lifestyle in 21 Days and Burn Fat - Includes Autophagy, OMAD, Meal Plan Content

Christine Moore

© Copyright 2019 - All rights reserved.

The content contained within this book may not be reproduced, duplicated or transmitted without direct written permission from the author or the publisher.

Under no circumstances will any blame or legal responsibility be held against the publisher, or author, for any damages, reparation, or monetary loss due to the information contained within this book. Either directly or indirectly.

<u>Legal Notice:</u>
This book is copyright protected. This book is only for personal use. You cannot amend, distribute, sell, use, quote or paraphrase any part, or the content within this book, without the consent of the author or publisher.

Disclaimer Notice:

Please note the information contained within this document is for educational and entertainment purposes only. All effort has been executed to present accurate, up to date, and reliable, complete information. No warranties of any kind are declared or implied. Readers acknowledge that the author is not engaging in the rendering of legal, financial, medical or professional advice. The content within this book has been derived from various sources. Please consult a licensed professional before attempting any techniques outlined in this book.

By reading this document, the reader agrees that under no circumstances is the author responsible for any losses, direct or indirect, which are incurred as a result of the use of information contained within this document, including, but not limited to, — errors, omissions, or inaccuracies.

Contents

Introduction _____ 1

Chapter 1:
Fundamentals of the Ketogenic Diet _____ 3

Chapter 2:
Ketosis _____ 26

Chapter 3:
Keto Nutritional Break Down _____ 34

Chapter 4:
Keto Meats and Nuts Products _____ 40

Chapter 5:
Keto Vegetable Products _____ 48

Chapter 6:
Keto Fruits, Dairy, and Oil Products _____ 53

Chapter 7:
Well Formulated Ketogenic Meals _____ 57

Chapter 8:
Finding Your Carb Sweet Spot _____ 60

Chapter 9: Intermittent Fasting	62
Chapter 10: Why Try Intermittent Fasting	75
Chapter 11: Keto and Intermittent Fasting	86
Chapter 12: Intermittent Fasting Regiments	91
Chapter 13: Beginners 4 Week Plan	97
Chapter 14: Big No No's	117
Chapter 15: Tips and Tricks and FAQs	121
Conclusion	140

POWERFUL Ketogenic DIET AND INTERMITTENT FASTING Secrets

COMPLETE KETO FAST GUIDE TO GAIN THE LOW-CARB CLARITY LIFESTYLE IN 21 DAYS AND BURN FAT - INCLUDES AUTOPHAGY, OMAD, MEAL PLAN CONTENT

CHRISTINE MOORE

Introduction

Beginning a new lifestyle can be daunting. It doesn't matter even if you know that the lifestyle promises many benefits such as weight loss and improved health without the drawbacks of crash or fad diets. A lifestyle change will impact your life, and you can be unsure on how to approach the change. But there is no need to fear. In this book, you will learn all you need to know about the Ketogenic diet, how to transition onto it fully within thirty days, manage any side effects, pair it with helpful exercises and intermittent fasting, and much more to get you well on your way toward success.

I have designed this book in a way that it is easy to understand the secrets of the Ketogenic diet, ketosis, and the countless health benefits associated with this lifestyle change alongside intermittent fasting. This whole book will help you shift to the Ketogenic world without any fears.

Ketogenic diets have been in use for thousands of years for their many health benefits, ease of implementation, and simply because of the environments we evolved in.

Powerful Ketogenic Diet and Intermittent Fasting Secrets

Even if you are a beginner to the diet, you will be able to adapt easily. Because this diet works to improve health while also decreasing weight, it has become a popular choice for everyone who wishes to lose weight, live a healthy lifestyle, or both. It is the best way to rapidly lose weight without sacrificing your health or taking harmful drugs.

The Ketogenic diet is very scientific in how it works. It is designed to put the body in a state of ketosis. You attain this state when your body starts burning fat stores for fuel, instead of sugars. As you can imagine, burning the storage of fat is exactly what you need to do to lose the type of weight that you want to lose, while maintaining your muscles.

Along with burning fat stores, ketosis has a neurological effect that will leave you feeling happier and less hungry. Both results will further help you lose any amount of weight you want. Because it is a healthy way to eat, you can continue with the Ketogenic diet indefinitely to maintain the ideal weight for your body type.

Chapter 1:
Fundamentals of the Ketogenic Diet

The word Ketogenic is getting a lot of hype these days and comes to the limelight more often than before. Since the whole diet plan of the book centers on a Ketogenic lifestyle, we will dive deeper to expand your understanding of the Ketogenic Diet.

Ketogenic diet refers to a group comprising many regimens that are known to contain low amounts of carbs with "high-fat, moderate protein" or "moderate fat, high-protein." The meaning of Keto originates from a metabolic process that occurs in the body called Ketosis. The process is essential in contributing toward the loss of that extra pound.

What is Ketosis? It is a healthy and natural metabolic process taking place in the body in which stored fat is burned to release some chemicals known as the Ketones. The ketones are essential in lowering fat levels in the human body and provide energy for various activities we undertake. When there is a scarcity of carbohydrate from the food you take, the fat in your body is burnt to provide that energy, which your carbs could not offer. Because of the process, production of ketones occurs. More will be explained later.

The Ketogenic diet involves high consumption of fats, a limited intake of proteins, and an almost limited intake of carbohydrates. The limited glucose intake can trigger satiety and allow you to attain a state of ketosis, which is the metabolism of fats for energy. This aids to hasten a healthy weight loss process without having to resort to starvation. Many may find this concept unappealing and questionable as there exists public knowledge linking fats as a cause of heart diseases. Moreover, skeptics do not believe its claim of getting rid of fatty deposits in the body by eating more fats as it is essentially fighting fire with fire.

The Ketogenic diet has become a wildly popular diet in recent years. However, the Ketogenic diet is not new. In fact, it has been in practice since the 1920s when it was originally created as a treatment for epilepsy. Also called "Keto," this diet focuses on changing eating habits to center on lower carb intake. The objective is to ensure that you ingest less than 50g of the net carbohydrates each day, not including carbs from fiber, so that the body can transition into a state of ketosis.

It is intended to make sure the body gets enough protein and nutrients to stay healthy and energized, but not so many that it gains weight.

Over the years, as the diet gained popularity, it began to be used for additional therapies, including the treatment of rare metabolic diseases, brain tumors, autism, depression, migraine headaches, and even Type 2 Diabetes. It has also been in extensive use for traumatic brain injuries, strokes, Parkinson's, and Alzheimer's disease. Oncologists even recommend this diet to cancer patients.

Many people struggling with weight issues and health conditions are always on the lookout for diets that can work for them and grant the desired results. Finding diets that can provide sustained results over long-term has been a challenge. Ketogenic diet is good for losing weight and to maintain a healthy lifestyle in the long-term. For a diet plan to be effective; it shouldn't be just capable of yielding the desired results; it should also be one that many find to be enjoyable.

When you have been eating in a given way for your entire life; finding instant changes when you start on a new diet such as the Ketogenic diet may not be automatic as the body takes time to completely shift and adapt to the new lifestyle. The human body was never designed to burn sugar for energy, going by human history. The craze about sugar is something that has been adopted recently however, even the ancestors lived their lives off meat and vegetables. The human bodies were designed to burn fat for fuel and the body has been proven to operate at optimum when utilizing fat for fuel.

Powerful Ketogenic Diet and Intermittent Fasting Secrets

Following a Ketogenic diet enables the body to burn fat for fuel which in turn accelerates weight loss alongside increased energy levels. Maintaining a healthy lifestyle is then possible without focusing much on restricting intake of calories, or even eating boring and bland meals to attain the desired results.

In a Ketogenic diet, you take high-fat and low-carb food for a longer period to start the process of ketosis in your body. You ingest protein in moderate. The reduction of carbohydrates in your body allows the already available fat to take its place.

When a person is on Ketogenic diet, the body gets to burn fat for fuel instead of burning sugar for fuel as it normally happens when one is on high carb diet. Being on this diet completely changes the functioning of the body but in quite a good way. It is based on the premise that the human body is designed to burn fat for energy instead of sugar.

When you consume foods that have high levels of carbs, the body gets to produce glucose and insulin. The body prefers use of glucose since the conversion of glucose molecule to energy is much easier. Insulin also gets produced to help with processing glucose to the bloodstream by transporting it all through the body. When glucose is utilized as the primary source of energy, the fats that gets consumed doesn't get utilized and instead ends up being stored in the body. Going by an average person's diet; glucose is normally the main source of energy. It may not bring much problem for the body especially when one is involved in high energy activities that ensure most of the energy that gets consumed is utilized.

A problem arises when the body produces more glucose than what is required. The extra glucose then gets converted to fat which then gets stored. Since the body utilizes glucose as the main source of energy, the glucose that gets converted to fat is never used. Whenever the body runs out of glucose, the brain sends signals that you want more glucose, so you are more likely to feel cravings for sugary things or a piece of snack. Being in such a cycle leads to development of a body that's not only overweight but also prone to several health-related diseases.

The process of carb reduction enhances the efficiency of your metabolic state known as ketosis. The fat starts burning faster and turns into ketones. These ketones provide more energy to enhance your mental power. Similarly, this diet also reduces the insulin and blood sugar content in your body. All in all, your body obtains multiple health benefits with a disciplined diet of Ketogenic.

Despite its benefits, the Ketogenic diet isn't for everybody. It requires strict tracking of your intake at the beginning to ensure that you're staying under the maximum of carbohydrates allowed (50 grams), which can be a deterrent to some. It's also not an easy diet to follow as it almost completely cuts off access to the comfort foods and cravings that we typically reach for. Basically, anything with refined sugar in it is a big "no."

Types of Keto

Standard Ketogenic Diet (SKD) – It is the type of Keto that has high-fats, low carbs and moderate protein each day. Standard percentages include 5% of carbs, 75% of fat, and about 20% of protein. The objective of the diet is to ensure that the body enters the state of ketosis to enable weight loss and decrease the frequency of epileptic seizures.

The diet does not allow the consumption of fruits, starches and milk. People feed on cheese, oils, butter and fatty meats. The diet allows carbs of under 30 grams. It is not advisable to work out when following the diet since there is not much energy due to fewer carbs ingested.

SKD is not good for individuals who work out regularly. It is good for sedentary people, obese people and those who are not willing to exercise. The diet is known to regulate hunger, controls intake of carbs and triggers fat loss process without the need of working out. You need to strictly follow for seven days consecutively.

When one consumes a low number of calories for a longer period, it may slow down metabolism which may prevent further weight loss. In the absence of occasional high carb in a diet, Ghrelin and Leptin (which are fat loss hormones) cannot be reset. You are advised not to stay on a diet for long.

After successful weight loss and you can work out, you can switch to the other Keto types which have more carbs that allow for more activity and will reset the Leptin and Ghrelin.

Targeted Ketogenic Diet (TKD) – The diet allows you to have an intake of carbs that range between 25 and 50 grams when you must work out. The carbs should be enough to sustain exercising without influencing ketosis. You have the option of working out three times a week. The targeted type of Ketogenic diet is decided by the workout you include. You can increase or decrease the carbohydrate content in your food depending on your workout's intensity.

Cyclical Ketogenic Diet (CKD) – The diet requires you to adhere to a strict version for five days and to binge on carbs for the remaining two days. Hence, the body smoothly converts the body fat into energy. It is easier to adhere to this type of diet since it allows you to have as many carbs as possible during the two days.

High Protein Ketogenic Diet: This one resembles the diet patterns of the standard type. However, you take about 35% of protein when following this Ketogenic diet. The fat portion stays 60%, while the carbs included are 5% only. Sports personalities, athletes, and bodybuilders utilize targeted and cyclical methods popularly.

History of Keto

Keto diet is a technique developed by modern physicians in the 1920's for treatment of epilepsy. The Keto diet is a high-fat diet with a moderate level of protein and low in carbohydrate in medicine used to treat epilepsy in children. The Ketogenic diet makes the human body to begin burning fats instead of carbohydrates. Keto diet therapy was developed as an alternative option for nonmainstream fasting. Doctors noticed that some epilepsy patients have exhibited signs of starving and some patients have low blood sugar. For many years, mankind new that fasting was geared towards the treatment of several diseases. This was studied in detail by ancient Indian physicians and ancient Greek physicians. An early discourse in the Hippocratic Corpus, "On the Sacred Disease," gives details how diet changes helped in management of epilepsy. In 1911, the first scientific study of fasting was used as a treatment for epilepsy in France. The experiment was conducted on twenty epileptic patients; all were detoxed by consuming a low-calorie vegetarian diet.

Advantages of Keto

Many people have claimed how being on Ketogenic diet changed their life and that's a fact that has been proven by many. Ketogenic diet is much more than a diet, it's a lifestyle that provides numerous benefits.

Weight Loss: One of the major motivations of being on Ketogenic diet is for weight loss. When on Ketogenic diet, the body uses fat as a source of energy and will then begin burning the unwanted fat which eventually leads to weight loss. Since the body can't take energy from carbs and sugars, the ketosis directs the system to draw energy from stored fat deposits and as you have guessed it, it gets this energy by burning these fat cells first. When on Keto diet, the level of fat storing hormone insulin drops, which then allows the fat cells to travel to the liver where it gets converted to ketones. The body eventually becomes a fat burning machine which makes weight loss to be much easier. Other than the ketosis process, a Keto diet can help you lose weight because of several reasons.

First, as opposed to processed snacks and other high carbohydrate foods, eating fat makes you eat less due to the effective satiating effect it induces on your metabolism. When you eat foods like cheese, fatty fish, avocado and nuts, the fat content gets into the intestines and triggers release of hormones. Such hormones among them are the cholecystokinin and Peptide YY to help control satiety and appetite and can make you feel fuller for longer. The satiating effect of fat is linked to its complexity in chemical composition that demands for a longer time to digest and extra energy to break down. A scientific study found out polyunsaturated fats, commonly referred to as "PUFAs," can trigger fullness to a bigger extent than meals with lower fatty acids. Eating a high-fat diet can also help you stick to your diet plan and in turn burn extra fat or lose weight.

Secondly, fat speeds up the rate of metabolism compared to a low-fat or high carb diet due to its link with fat burning hormones called adipokines. Hormones such as adiponectin are formed from fat cells and their work is to boost the rate at which fats are metabolized. To further explain the importance of eating fats, a study found out that eating healthier fat can help speed up metabolism and reduce storage of visceral or belly fat. Findings in this study showed that people who consumed high-fat foods burned 300 more calories daily compared to the low-fat group. Better still, the high-fat group had a normal amount of blood insulin and was less likely to develop related diabetic conditions. The high-fat group fed on 60 percent fats, 30 percent proteins and only 10 percent carbs while the low-fat group consumed 60 percent carbs, 20 percent fats and 20 percent proteins.

In addition, fat acts as a solvent for fat-soluble nutrients such as vitamin A, D, E, and K. The body needs to absorb such nutrients to facilitate various metabolic functions, and deficiency of these nutrients can be detrimental. Insufficient amounts of vital minerals and vitamins may result in problems such as blood clots, blindness, brittle bones among others. For weight loss, you need vitamin D, as it helps metabolize body fat from regions such as the abdomen.

Controls Blood Sugar: when one is on a high carbohydrate diet; the body reaches a state where it's unable to handle the higher levels of insulin in the body. A person is then more likely to develop medical conditions such diabetes and increased blood sugar levels. When a person switches to a low carb diet, the blood sugar levels gets lowered which makes Ketogenic diet suitable for those with diabetes type 2. The diet also enables people to maintain consistent levels of blood sugar and overall improvement of health.

Mental Focus: it's not easy to understand how being on a high carb diet leads to having a cloudy way of thinking until you are off the diet. Mental focus is one of the major benefits that come with being on a Ketogenic diet. The diet that you are on has a substantial effect on your state of mental health as the brain requires almost 25% of the calories consumed to be able to execute various activities. The increased fat intake when you are on a Ketogenic diet helps in improving the functioning of the brain in various ways. Being on a diet that's not balanced leads to lack of mental clarity and that is likely to show up as having difficulty in remembering things, feelings of a foggy brain and inability to stay focused.

Ketones provide the body with a source of energy that enables it to process efficiently the extra glutamate into GABA and eventually decreases then reduces stimulation and improved mental focus. Most of the brain tissue consists of fatty acids so being on a high-fat diet leads to improved mental focus. The essential fatty acids such as omega-6 and omega-3 are very crucial for brain health. Being on Ketogenic diet also improves one's memory. Being on ketosis state helps in production of mitochondria and eventually increases the brain's memory cells.

Increased Levels of Energy: Being on Ketogenic diet brings to end feelings of fatigue naturally. You will then realize that you have a clearer mind with better moods. Most of the high carb and traditional diets are centered around foods that are sugary and have starchy carbs. These carbs normally spike and increase levels of insulin in the body which eventually results into high blood sugar levels. A rapid rise in levels of insulin also causes sluggishness and increased feelings of lethargy.

Once a person shifts to a low carb, high-fat diet, they also get to experience increased levels of energy, less compulsive eating and cravings for carbs, and better mental concentration. With increased feelings of alertness and less need for sleep also come increased levels of energy.

Reduce Triglycerides: Triglycerides are a certain type of fat present in the blood. Once food is consumed, the body converts the food into glucose with the excess calories being converted into triglycerides for storage in the body cells. Being on a high carb diet increases the level of triglycerides which then gets reduced when one shifts to low carb diet. Reduced levels also lower chances of contracting ailments.

Reduced Cholesterol: consumption of high carb foods has the potential of increasing levels of cholesterol in the body with great chances of causing heart disease or stroke. There is the high-density lipoprotein (HDL) which is also known as the good cholesterol and the low-density lipoprotein (LDL) also referred to as the bad cholesterol. LDL is known to transport cholesterol present in the liver and other body parts which then creates a buildup around the arteries. HDL is involved in the carrying of cholesterol from other parts of the body to the liver where they get utilized or excreted out of the body. Being on Ketogenic diet reduces the level of bad cholesterol which then results into reduced risks of heart disease and other ailments.

Treatment for Metabolic Syndrome: this is a medical condition that's associated with the risk of heart disease and diabetes. The condition consists of a collection of symptoms such as the ones below;

- Abdominal obesity
- High triglycerides
- Low HDL levels
- High levels of blood sugar
- Elevated blood pressure

Improved Digestion: Improved digestion depends on the health of the gut as over 70% of the immune system is found in the gut. A high carb diet tends to release sugar, antibiotics, additives, and pesticides that affect the good bacteria required along the intestinal tract for efficient digestion. A shift to Ketogenic diet enables the body to burn fat for fuel which results into production of more good bacteria while eliminating the bad bacteria. The result is an improved digestive system.

Treating Gastrointestinal Problems: digestive issues like irritable bowel syndrome, acid reflux, gallstones, inflammation, bloating, heartburn can lead to chronic diseases if not controlled. A change in your diet can fix all this. Keto diet helps in improving your eating habits and reduces the discomfort caused due to an irritable gut.

Epilepsy Control: The Keto diet has been utilized for nearly a century to help treat patients suffering from seizures and Epilepsy. Even to this day, it is widely used by major health clinics e.g. Mayo Clinic to treat kids and young adults suffering from the disease. While it can't cure Epilepsy (which has no cure to this day), it can certainly help control the number of medications needed to control Epilepsy symptoms and ease inflammation of the nervous system.

Acne and Eczema: another health benefit of the Keto diet, which not many people are aware of, is helping ease acne and eczema breakouts, as well as other inflammatory skin disorders (dermatitis, scalp issues). The Keto diet can do this by decreasing inflammation inside the body and encouraging tissue cells to repair themselves faster and more effectively than before. It appears to have the opposite effect of following high-carb and high-sugar diets, which have been found to indirectly cause acne and skin inflammation in general.

Reduced Risk of Heart Disease: A Ketogenic diet helps in regulating the levels of blood sugar and lowers the blood pressure levels. Since it is a low-carb and high-fat diet, it leads to a reduction of triglycerides and cholesterol. This is because of the increase in the levels of HDL (good cholesterol) while reducing the levels of LDL (bad cholesterol). A high level of HDL indicates a lower risk of cardiac diseases.

Improves Women's Health: A Keto diet helps in strengthening fertility. Polycystic Ovarian Syndrome is a widespread hormonal disorder in women, and it can be treated and controlled by following the Keto diet. This diet also helps in overcoming other symptoms like acne and obesity. It regularizes the menstrual cycle as well.

Strengthens the Eyes: increased amounts of sugar in an individual's system can be toxic and can deteriorate eyesight. This increases the risk of cataracts, and a diet that drastically cuts down on sugar reduces such risks as well.

Controls Appetite: hunger pangs can make many individuals give up on a certain diet. A Keto diet is rich in fats, and this makes you feel fuller for longer, in a healthy way. Unintentionally, your calorie intake reduces too.

Dangers of the Ketogenic Diet

Keto diet is a safe diet plan, but it may lead to some side effects. I think I should let you know that there are some changes which you might face during the early days of your Keto diet due to changes in your body's overall homeostatic functions.

There are a few different side-effects of the Ketogenic diet that you should be aware of. Some of them might be uncomfortable or annoying at first, but they are temporary. You just need to stick with the diet for a week or so before you see some improvement.

However, these symptoms will eventually go away! So, don't be alarmed if you face any of such symptoms like aggravation, Keto-Flu and Mental Fogginess among other explained below.

Physical Performance: one the main side effects of the Ketogenic diet is a temporary lull in physical performance. You might see some limitations when you first begin this diet, but as the body adapts and adjusts to using fat as its primary source of fuel, all your endurance and strength will return.

Effect on Liver, Muscles and Frequent Urination: carbohydrate is stored in our bodies mainly in the liver and muscles in the form of glycogen. An individual requires approximately 600 calories to sustain daily without eating anything. But if you are not into too much of exercising and have been leading a sedentary life most of your life, the carbohydrate starts to accumulate. On the other hand, if you exercise rigorously and your carb intake is low, you will have exhausted the glycogen very soon. But at the same time, you experience fatigue and tend to get dehydrated, which is not good for your health. Since there is little carbohydrate left and you carry on with the normal daily activities, you gradually get dehydrated. So, if you are opting for Ketogenic diet, you ought to do away with rigorous exercise and intense weight training.

After the first day or two of the diet, you'll most likely notice that you're making some more frequent trips to the bathroom. Your body is burning up those extra glycogen stores in the liver and muscles. Breaking down the glycogen will release a lot of water. As your carbohydrate intake and your glycogen stores decrease, your kidneys are going to begin getting rid of this excess water.

In addition, as the levels of insulin circulating through your body lower, your kidneys will begin excreting some excess sodium, which is going to cause more frequent urination. This side effect will eventually cease.

Risk of Cancer: if you are on a low carbohydrate diet, and if you are not able to maintain it properly with the right number of elements, you will have trouble with digestion and lead to bowel and constipation irregularities. This makes you susceptible to cardiovascular diseases and digestive cancer. Also, another cause of concern is that if you deprive yourself of legume, fruits, vegetables, and grains, it results in insufficient intake of potassium, vitamin C, and antioxidants. Also, intake of phytonutrients is compromised.

Prone to Heart Disease: there are a few categories of high-fat food items that include egg yolks, coconut, and lard. These have a high saturated fat content but low carbohydrate as well as protein content. Consuming this kind of food over a long period of time makes you susceptible to heart diseases. Also, it has been observed that a diet high in fat content have a detrimental effect on the brain cells. This is because there is a set of brain cells that regulate body weight.

Dizziness and Fatigue: as you begin getting rid of water, you're going to lose some minerals such as potassium, salt, and magnesium. Lower levels of these minerals can cause lightheadedness, dizziness, and fatigue. It can also cause headaches, muscle cramps and skin itchiness.

To reduce these side effects, consume enough replacement minerals. Consume more sea salt and drink some salty broth. In addition, eat foods high in minerals, such as leafy green vegetables and avocados.

If your carbohydrate consumption is lower than sixty carbohydrates per day, you'll need to carry on eating a moderate amount of salt. However, if you are under high blood pressure medication, you need to check with a doctor first.

In addition, you might want to take a magnesium supplement of 400mg before bed every night. If you have heart or kidney conditions, check with a doctor before taking this dose.

It's also important to eat at least two cups of raw, green leafy vegetables each day. These provide you with vitamin K and potassium and will help greatly with hunger cravings.

Low Blood Sugar (Hypoglycemia): with a higher carbohydrate diet, the body releases insulin to convert carbs to glucose. When you abruptly decrease that carbohydrate intake on the Ketogenic diet plan, you might have some fleeting low blood sugar incidents.

Headaches: as your body adapts to the ketosis, headaches can come about for a few different reasons. You could feel lightheaded and feel like you have the flu for a few days. This is usually due to mineral deficiencies. To see if it's from sodium, try putting a quarter of a teaspoon of salt into a glass of water and drink it. You should feel better in about twenty minutes.

Increase your salt and water intake to reduce headache symptoms. These should improve after few days. If not, add a few more carbohydrates to your daily total.

Constipation: usually the same cause as frequent urination, salt loss. Can also be caused by magnesium imbalances or excess nuts or dairy consumption. The intake of magnesium supplement of 400mg will help with this. If 400mg of magnesium citrate doesn't help, then you might want to cut back on how much dairy you consume in order to balance out your calcium intake. Drinks tons of water and monitor nut and dairy consumption.

Sugar Cravings: this is very common. People may laugh, but sugar cravings can be just as bad as any other addictive product. As your body goes through the process of burning fat rather than sugar, there is a two to twenty-one-day period where carbohydrate cravings can be quite intense. If you can wait it out, then the cravings will disappear. Be strong! Eating a huge amount of carbohydrates will bring those cravings right back, and halt ketosis. For some people, eating sugar in any amount starts the process all over again.

Diarrhea: this isn't an unusual side effect of a low carbohydrate diet, and it should resolve after a few days. This can result from eating too much protein and not enough fat. Eating a high protein, low carbohydrate, low-fat diet causes symptoms that are known as rabbit starvation. Be sure you replace the carbohydrates you cut out of your diet with more fat.

Weakness or Shakiness: this is one of the side effects of the hypoglycemia you can experience. It's also a symptom of low amounts of minerals in your system. Add a little more protein to your diet and eat more salt. In addition, include more foods with potassium. You can also take a 99mg potassium citrate supplement to help offset this symptom.

Muscle Cramps: this is another side effect of losing minerals, especially magnesium. Take three slow release magnesium tablets for twenty days, and then continue to take one tablet each day after twenty days.

Sleeping Problems: some individuals report difficulty sleeping while following the Keto Diet. This may indicate low serotonin or insulin levels. Try eating a snack that has protein and a little carbohydrate right before you go to bed. The carbohydrates release insulin, which lets more tryptophan from the protein you consumed get into the brain. This is a precursor to serotonin, which has an overall calming effect.

Sleep problems may also be caused by histamine intolerance. Low carbohydrates foods often contain high amounts of histamines, and some people will react to a higher intake of these types of foods with sleeplessness and anxiety.

Kidney Stones: some people bring this side effect up when they try to convince people that a low carbohydrate diet is dangerous. They base this on reports of calcium-based kidney stones reported by physicians who used the Ketogenic diet for children who had epilepsy. However, this is not a very accurate comparison.

First, the diet that is given to children with epilepsy contains close to 90% fat and processed powders that are used to make shakes used a lot for children who have epilepsy. A real Ketogenic food diet is different and includes more protein. However, if you're worried about it, a citrate supplement can minimize your risk.

Lowered T3 Thyroid Hormones: while this side effect is usually viewed as negative, it's a natural result of a ketosis lower calorie diet. The same thing happens on calorie-restricted high carbohydrate diets.

In addition, it's possible your body becomes more sensitive to the T3 when you're in ketosis state, as your body requires less of this hormone to get the job done.

Racing Heart or Heart Palpitations: some people experience heart palpitations when they begin a Keto diet or after they've been on one for a few weeks or months. It's been reported this is more likely to happen if the person has a low blood pressure normally. There are a few other potential factors that may cause heart palpitations.

Nutrient Deficiency - A multivitamin that has the RDA for selenium and zinc, as well as a magnesium supplement, is strongly recommended. You can also try some homemade bone broth.

Insulin Resistance - transient hypoglycemia can result from not eating often enough or not eating enough fat and protein.

Electrolyte imbalance or Dehydration - Making some mineral water at home and drinking a cup in the morning and one in the evening can help if this is your problem. In addition, be sure you consume plenty of water to avoid dehydration.

Too much MCT or Coconut Oil - As you add these to your diet, begin with small amounts and increase them over time. Never rely on coconut oil as your only fat intake. Be sure you include other fats, such as ghee, butter, animal fats, and olive oil, too.

Hair Loss: although rare, some people report experiencing accelerated hair loss while following the Keto diet. This is not related directly to the Ketogenic diet but is associated with a change in diet. This process is known as telogen effluvium, a medical term for hair loss due to a change in hormone levels or metabolism. Ketogenic diets create a lower insulin level, which is one of the main hormones in the human body, and hair loss can be a natural but temporary side effect.

Remember, these are potential side effects. You may experience these side effects, you may not! However, it is good to be prepared for what potential effects to expect. These side effects are temporary. Once your body adjusts to the diet, they should subside.

Chapter 2:
Ketosis

As the carbohydrate is reduced in the human body, it starts utilizing the available fat as fuel. The whole body starts to get energy from fat only. Ketosis is a metabolic state that gets induced when the body begins to use fats as the main source of fuel instead of carbohydrates. The body while in such a metabolic process gets to break down the stored fats as source of energy instead of glucose since the body is deprived of enough carbs that can be converted into glucose. The reason for being on Ketogenic diet is so that the body can get into a metabolic state which is referred to as ketosis. The event of ketosis occurs in your body during strict diet or fasting conditions.

In terms of health benefits, ketosis offers quick loss of weight, increased performance level of the body, and improved health condition of the heart. However, excessive ketosis can prove to be harmful to certain diabetic patients.

Ketogenic diet is an effective way to maximize the process of ketosis. Regular high-fat and low-carbohydrate diet helps in replacing the glucose with the ketone molecules. Hence, all the body fat burns simultaneously as you take them. As a result, your body starts losing weight, which you can control according to your weight goals.

Ketosis is principally dependent on the bodily levels of three essential components: glucagon, insulin and blood glucose. The entire process starts and ends with metabolism.

As mentioned above, the body breaks down ingested substances to use as fuel for the body; namely carbohydrates, fats, and proteins (in that order). When the primary source is about to run dry, the body moves on to the substance that is second in line and, when this too has a low supply, it uses the tertiary choice.

Under normal circumstances, blood glucose levels are kept within a healthy range by insulin. It does so by facilitating the transport of glucose from the bloodstream into body cells. If the pancreas fails to produce an adequate amount of insulin, there would be an unmanageable and potentially harmful level of glucose in the blood.

Glucagon, on the other hand, is considered as the "antagonistic hormone" of insulin. This substance, which is also secreted by the pancreas, is produced when insulin levels fall low. Such a situation emanates inadequate consumption of carbohydrates and meal-skipping. It works by turning the glycogen present in the liver into a simpler form - glucose. However, if this process goes on until there is a depletion of glycogen supply in the liver, the pancreas will begin to break down lipids (also known as fatty acids) into ketone bodies to use as energy. This secondary means of fueling the body is known as ketosis.

How Ketosis Works

When the level of glycogen and glucose are depleted in the body; the levels of insulin and blood sugar also gets to decrease, and the body is then forced to look for alternative energy source. The body then begins to break down the stored fats for energy through a process that's referred to as beta-oxidation, which leads to increased levels of acetoacetate. Acetoacetate then forms the ketone body that gets transported through the blood and to the brain for provision of energy.

When the body produces enough ketones with significant levels of over 0.5mM in the blood, it's already in ketosis state. One of the fastest ways of getting the body to ketosis is through fasting. When the body is deprived of food, it automatically switches to utilizing the stored fats for energy. When getting started on a Ketogenic diet, beginners can consider engaging in periods of fasting so that the body gets to switch to ketosis state much faster.

One of the common misconceptions associated with being on a high carb diet is that the brain needs carbs to be able to function effectively. The truth is that the brain happily burns ketones and intake of carbs may not be necessary at all. To attain the metabolic state of ketosis, foods should be consumed in the ratio of 75% or more of fats, 20% or less of proteins and 5% or less of carbohydrates. There are plenty of foods that you can choose from at every meal to be able to reach the required macronutrients ratios.

How do You Know You Are in Ketosis?

There are technical and general ways to find out and ensure that you are in ketosis. You can get your blood samples tested, or the same with urine samples as well as breath samples. Generally, there are visible signs that tell you that you have successfully achieved ketosis:

Increased Desire for Drinking Water: Dry mouth is a common sign that you are going through ketosis. The desire for drinking water increases due to that. This happens because your body asks for electrolytes. People using Ketogenic diet are recommended 2 cups of bouillon every day along with large quantities of water.

Fruity Smell: Incredible right? The production of ketones also creates acetone as the by-product in the cells. This acetone comes out when you exhale. Hence, the breath gives a fruity smell. It generally smells like a flavored nail polish. The similar smell is possible when you sweat, especially during an intense workout. However, the fruity breath stays only for a little while.

Increased Urge of Urination: During the initial period of Ketogenic diet, you can experience an increased urge for urination. The creation of ketones in your body also sends some acetoacetate to your urine. The consistent creation of ketones increases the level of urine generation as well. Hence, you end up in the bathroom more than usual. It is the same acetoacetate that helps in assuring the level of ketosis with a urine sample test.

Higher Energy Level: If you can cross the initial low phase of the Keto diet, the rest of the experience makes you feel highly energetic. The initial low feeling is also called the Keto flu, which stays for the initial period of the diet. As the body starts utilizing fat for fuel, you get your energy level back. In fact, the produced ketones further enhance the activeness of your brain cells. Hence, you can think better and make decisions faster.

Reduction in Hunger: The fat stored in your body begins to provide regular energy for the body. Once the cycle is created, your body declines the need for food. Hence, many Keto diet followers inform about the reduction in hunger level. This also generates the condition of fasting and further increases the weight loss activity.

Heart Palpitations: You may begin to feel 'fluttery' as a result of dehydration or because of an insufficient intake of salt. Try to adjust, but if you don't feel better quickly, you should seek emergency care.

Disrupted Sleep: The restless night is also a typical side effect. Vitamin supplements can sometimes remedy the problem that can be caused by a lowered insulin and serotonin level. For a quick fix; try 1/2 of a tablespoon of fruit spread and a square of chocolate.

Induction Flu: The diet can make you irritable, nauseous, a bit confused or lethargic, and possibly suffer from a headache. Several days into the plan should remedy these effects. If not, add 1/2 teaspoon of salt to a glass of water, and drink it to help with the side effects. You may need to do this once a day for about the first week, and it could take about 15 to 20 minutes before it helps. It will go away!

Leg Cramps: The loss of magnesium (a mineral) can be a demon and create a bit of pain with the onset of the Keto diet plan changes. With the loss of the minerals during urination, you could experience bouts of cramps in your legs.

Constipation: During the Ketogenic plan, you must drink plenty of water. You can quickly become constipated because of dehydration. The low carbs contribute to the issue. Eat the right veggies and add a small amount of salt to your food to help with the movements. If all else fails, try some Milk of Magnesia.

Checking Ketone Levels

In order to achieve ketosis, you need to have serum ketones between 0.5 and 3.0mM. Below are easy to use home kits to know your ketone levels.

Blood Ketone Meter: It serves as the best and most accurate technique of measuring Beta-Hydroxybutyrate. Blood ketone meters can determine, with precision, the level of ketones in the blood; however, they are quite expensive. The meter costs around $40 and each test strip costs $5. This means that if you want to measure your ketone levels daily, you will need to part with $50.

Breathalyzer: As mentioned earlier, when on a Ketogenic diet, your breath has a distinct smell. A Breathalyzer is a cheap way to measure the concentration of acetone. Keep in mind though that breath ketones can vary from blood ketones.

Urine Test / Urine Ketone Strips: This is one way to measure your ketones for the purpose of ascertaining whether you are in ketosis. Using urine strips, you can easily and simply determine your ketosis without much cost. Testing your urine will readily reveal to you if you have gone over the roof top by eating higher than recommended carbs. Once you dip the stick into your urine, it will turn purple indicating the presence of ketones in your body. A good result for the presence of ketones is dark purple color. When no precise color is shown, it means that you might not have entered ketosis yet.

Ketosis and other urine detection strips may not be as effective because they only show the excess ketone bodies being excreted from the body through the urine. However, they are easy to use and affordable.

Observation: It is possible to know you have attained ketosis by taking a moment listening to the body. For instance, when in ketosis, your breath, urine and sweat smell of acetone, which is a "fruity" smell. If you detect this, then you are most likely in ketosis.

Christine Moore

With that understanding of what happens to your body during ketosis, the question you may want to ask is; how then do you get started on the diet?

Chapter 3:
Keto Nutritional Break Down

Being in ketosis is all dependent on consuming the right types of nutrients, the right amounts, and eating those nutrients from the right sources. Let's start with the right types of nutrients. The foods we eat are categorized into different "macronutrients" (more casually known as "macros" if you want to freshen-up your food lingo!). The three main macros are carbs, protein, and fat. If you want to reach Ketosis, then you really need to pay close attention to your macros. Too many carbs and you'll blow your chances, too many proteins and you can really slow the process or stop it all together.

For those of you who've been on the Keto Diet for even a few months, it is clear why these three nutrients are important. They each provide nutrition and energy to your cells that you can't get without consuming them.

1. Carbs
Carbohydrates are most commonly recognized as "starchy" foods such as bread, pasta, potatoes, and rice. However, carbohydrates include sugars and sugar-containing foods such as fruit, candy, cakes,

alcohol... you name it. When you ingest carbs, the body turns them into glucose (blood sugar), which is then used for energy. As soon as the amount of sugar in the blood is raised, your pancreas gets the message to pump out more insulin, so the blood sugar can be processed and moved around the body as energy.

2. Protein

Together with the good fats, protein is one of your body's primary sources of fuel! You can either eat animal proteins, such as meat, fish, eggs, and seafood, or plant protein that's found in nuts, beans, and quinoa. Your brain requires massive amounts of protein for all its processing and daily functions. Protein is very similar to a general handyman, repairing and rebuilding your tissues, making enzymes for better digestion, making hormones (which is what it also does in your brain), and contributes towards building many new cells in your body for things like your muscles, skin, blood, cartilage, and bones. Together with being a fuel source, you can see why it's very important for your body.

3. Fat

Fat is the most important Macro on the Keto Diet, and the most misunderstood, falsely accused, misaligned, and just plain hated. "Fat" is just a short-term nickname for the fatty acids that are present in fats. Fatty acids are long chains of molecules with different chemical components that are various combinations of three atoms: carbon, hydrogen, and oxygen.

There are two types of fats that are lurking in the foods present at your grocery store or served at restaurants:

- *Good Fats*
- *Bad Fats*

Basically, the good fats give you amazing energy, improve your good cholesterol, benefit insulin levels, and control your blood sugar. The bad fats do the opposite. They contribute towards weight gain, raise your bad LDL cholesterol levels, create inflammation, block your arteries, and contribute towards other chronic conditions.

How do you know which fat is your friend and which is your enemy? Read on below to tell the difference.

Good Fats

Saturated Fats – The fatty acid molecules are saturated with hydrogen atoms, thus giving these good fats their name. You can find saturated fats in animal products like meats and dairy. On the Keto Diet, you want to be consuming naturally occurring saturated fats from animals only.

Monounsaturated Fats – These fatty acids only have one double bond that links carbon atoms to hydrogen atoms. These fats don't have as many calories as the saturated fats, so you'd want to eat more of them. They do protect against cardiovascular disease though. Saturated fats come from animal sources, while monounsaturated fats come from plant sources – nuts, avocados, olive oil, etc.

Natural Polyunsaturated Fats – The processed version of these fatty acids is very bad for you, but the naturally occurring version is great! They're called different names like Omega-3 and Omega-6 fatty acids. You can get your Omega-3 and Omega-6 from walnuts, spinach, eggs, chia seeds, salmon, broccoli, and pumpkin seeds. All those foods are Keto Diet friendly, so eat up!

Bad Fats

Processed Saturated Fats – In addition to naturally occurring saturated fats, these fats can also be created in a laboratory and put into processed foods. That's why they go on the naughty list. Only get your saturated fats from animal sources like meat, dairy, eggs, and seafood.

Processed Polyunsaturated Fats – The natural version is good, but the processed polyunsaturated fats aren't good. If you avoid corn oil, soybean oil, margarine, and those types of foods, you won't be consuming these bad fats. That's why it is important to only buy Ketogenic Diet friendly ingredients and leave these bad fat sources on the shelf.

Trans Fats – Trans-fatty acids are the worst kinds of fats! These are the bad apples that spoil the bunch, because there are so many sources of good fats. But you've got to stay away from these ones.

They were created by the food industry and aren't found naturally occurring in sources from animals or plants. They're like a Frankenstein laboratory experiment gone wrong! If you eat even a small amount of trans fats, your bad cholesterol levels will rise, and you'll be more prone to disease. Trans fats are mostly found in fried or processed foods. Beware!

Fats which are "whole" or "from the source" such as eggs, grass-fed meats, heavy cream, butter, fresh fatty fish such as salmon are all healthy sources of fat. Products which have been processed and refined down to a "different" form than how they started are "bad" fats such as: margarine and vegetable oils (apart from olive oil).

A typical Keto diet, also known as a "long-chain triglyceride diet" usually ensures a consumption ratio of about 3 to 4 grams of fat for every 1 gram of carbohydrate and protein.

In order to ensure you are taking in the accurate levels of each macro, you should track your daily nutrient levels. The general rule is that your daily food should fit within these macro guidelines:

- Fats: 75% of your daily calories

- Protein: 20% of your daily calories

- Carbs: 5% of your daily calories

You may be wondering, what is the timeframe for one to enter ketosis? After 2 days of consuming 20 grams of carbs or less, most people will enter ketosis. Time taken may be, depending on body type, diet plan, and timing of eating.

If you are curious to know about how you can maximize your efforts to fully boost up your Ketosis levels, then all you need to do is follow these simple guidelines.

- Keep your daily carbohydrate intake below 20 carbs.

- Keep your protein levels at around 70g per day.

- Don't starve! Swallow adequate level of fat. Remember that the body is going to need fat to burn fat.

- Try to avoid snack times and stick to your breakfast, lunch and dinner meals with nothing in between.

Chapter 4:
Keto Meats and Nuts Products

You know that you can enjoy beef, bacon, chicken, lamb, cheese, and butter on the Ketogenic diet. So, in this portion, we are going to look at some of the animal-based products that need more recognition for their health benefits.

Sardines are tasty and accessible. If you want a quick meal, you simply must take a can off the shelf and warm it up in the oven for five minutes. Despite this, many people often reach for other canned fish, such as tuna instead. But, while tuna may have its benefits, you are greatly missing out on sardines. One of the great things about sardines is that because they are so small, they eat plankton and no other smaller fish. This leads to them having much less heavy metal toxicity and mercury than fish such as tuna. These fish are a great source of antioxidants, selenium, magnesium, calcium, iron, phosphorous, niacin, vitamin B12, vitamin D, and omega-3s. This leads to sardines being able to help lower cholesterol, increase metabolism, treat gum disease, lower inflammation, improve mental health, strengthen bones, increase energy, and more.

Liver from chicken, beef, duck, and other animals used to be quite popular in order not to waste food. But with the use of supermarkets and the ability to buy select cuts of meat, liver has largely fallen out of favor in America. This is disappointing since it contains many nutrients and health benefits. In fact, the number of nutrients in this small product is amazing. Some of the most potent nutrients within the liver are iron, vitamin B12, vitamin A, riboflavin, copper, choline, and folate.

This simple piece of meat can boost the immune system, increase eye health, increase cellular health and functioning, prevent anemia, increase heart and kidney health, promote the growth of new healthier cells, increase brain function, improve the absorption of iron, boost liver health, and increase energy.

Salmon may not be underappreciated, but many Americans still do not eat enough of this vital fish. Salmon is one of the healthiest fishes and one of the healthiest foods of any type to eat. One of the reasons for this is the large amount of omega-3 fatty acids within salmon. When purchasing salmon, it is best to get wild-caught when possible. This is because farm-raised salmon contains less omega-3s than wild-caught. Studies have found that by eating as little as two servings of salmon a week, we can reach the minimum amount of omega-3 needs.

Salmon is also high in many important B vitamins, selenium, potassium, and antioxidants. It has been found to help lower inflammation, reduce weight, protect against heart disease, protect brain health, and more.

Nuts are a wonderful part of the Ketogenic diet for people without allergies. But it is important to understand how they fit in. Otherwise, it could be easy to cause a stall in your weight loss. While nuts are high in nutrients and much higher in fats than carbs, it's important to realize that their carb count does add up. In fact, cashews, chestnuts, and pistachios are all too high in net carbs to be eaten on the Ketogenic diet. This is especially true because nuts add up quickly. While only an ounce is the serving, people often eat much more than this at any one time. But if you keep an eye on your serving size and how frequently you are eating nuts, you should be fine. However, if you do experience a stall in weight loss for multiple weeks in a row, you might want to cut back on nuts and dairy.

There are many reasons to enjoy pecans. One of the reasons is because they are the lowest nut in net carbs with an ounce containing only 1.1 net carbs. But there are other reasons as well. Pecans are not only the highest nut in antioxidants, but the USDA has even ranked it within the top fifteen antioxidant-rich foods. You can also receive many vitamins and minerals from these nuts, such as selenium, iron, manganese, calcium, zinc, magnesium, and potassium.

Pecans are high in oleic acid, the same type of fat within olives and avocados that give them their signature heart health promoting effect. They can improve digestion, lower cholesterol, reduce the risk of breast and colon cancer, boost the immune system, lower inflammation, treat skin conditions, and slow down aging.

Brazil nuts are a great source of vitamin E, certain B vitamins, magnesium, calcium, and zinc. But what they are best known for is their amazingly high concentration of selenium. In fact, these nuts are the highest known source of this vital nutrient. This micronutrient is an antioxidant and mineral that we require for hormone and immune health, and it helps to protect both our nervous system and cells. Selenium deficiency is well known to be a cause of hyperthyroidism and even sometimes mood disorders such as depression and anxiety. But, by supplementing your diet with natural sources of selenium, you may be able to manage the symptoms or completely recover from these conditions. Eating as few as five or six Brazil nuts can provide you with a full day's serving of selenium.

Macadamia nuts, while may be called a nut, are a seed. But, nonetheless, this nut contains a surprising number of health-promoting monounsaturated fats, magnesium, potassium, selenium, manganese, zinc, calcium, iron, B vitamins, and fiber. One of the types of fat in macadamia nuts is palmitoleic acid. This type of fat is an omega 7, which is incredibly rare but has many benefits. For instance, around our neurons, we have a protective fatty coating, known as myelin.

When this myelin begins to become damaged, it leads to symptoms of neurodegenerative diseases and mental illness. But, palmitoleic acid is a major component of our myelin, meaning that by eating more through macadamia nuts can promote our neurological health. As if that weren't enough to boost our brain, their contents of thiamine, copper, and iron are all essential for brain health.

Walnuts have long been centered in medical research for their many amazing properties. In fact, every year there is a medical conference at the University of California detailing all the latest research on this powerful nut. There is a good reason to choose walnuts; they are higher in antioxidant activity and omega-3 fats than any of the other nuts. The antioxidants from the plant compounds, vitamin E, and melatonin have many benefits, including lowering bad cholesterol and improving heart health. With the high number of omega-3s in walnuts, you can gain two and a half grams for each one-ounce serving.

The plant compounds within walnuts, known as polyphenols, have many benefits. One of these benefits is that they directly target inflammation and oxidative damage that is the direct cause of many illnesses. This means that they can directly impact cancer, Alzheimer's disease, diabetes, autoimmune diseases, neurological diseases, and more. Studies have also found that by consuming walnuts regularly, we may be able to lower high blood pressure.

Hazelnuts, also known as filberts, like many nuts are high in healthy fats and antioxidants. This nut has specifically been the focus of many studies on inflammation and how it leads to disease. In study after study, it has found that the antioxidants within hazelnuts, known as phenolic compounds, can greatly reduce inflammation. This, in turn, can help protect against cancer, neurodegenerative diseases, and more. Although, it's important to know that most of the antioxidants found within hazelnuts are within the skin of the nut. Not only that, but by roasting the nut prior to eating it, the number of antioxidants is reduced. Therefore, it is best to enjoy these nuts raw and with the skin intact.

Almonds may be higher in nuts than the others we have discussed so far, but they are still low enough to be eaten in moderation on the Ketogenic diet. In fact, products such as almond milk make a wonderful addition when you are on a Keto lifestyle. These nuts are high in vitamin E, manganese, phosphorus, calcium, iron, magnesium, antioxidants, and fiber. They have been shown to manage blood pressure, lower cholesterol, improve heart health, increase brain health, and promote strong bones and teeth.

Chia seeds are a small black seed that only recently took the world by storm due to their powerful nutrients. But despite only recently coming into the focus of health-conscious people, these seeds have a long and rich history with the Mayans and Aztecs. Part of the reason these seeds are so amazing is that despite their tiny size, they hold an incredible amount of nutrients. In fact, a single ounce of chia seeds contains only one-hundred and thirty-seven calories and two net carbs. This means that calorie for calorie, chia seeds are one of the best nutrient sources in the world. A few of the nutrients these seeds contain are phosphorous, manganese, zinc, B vitamins, magnesium, potassium, and omega-3 fatty acids. Of course, they also hold quite a few antioxidants, as well. In a single ounce of chia, you can also gain four grams of protein and eight grams of healthy fats.

These seeds can help with weight loss, improve heart health, strengthen bones, lower inflammation levels, balance blood sugar, and more.

While sesame seeds may be tiny and overlooked, they are a rich source of healthy fats, antioxidants, fiber, magnesium, iron, calcium, potassium, phosphorous, zinc, copper, vitamin E, and certain B vitamins. These seeds have been shown to improve heart health, reduce the risk of certain cancers, prevent diabetes, increase bone strength, reduce male infertility, manage blood pressure, increase heart health, reduce inflammation, treat respiratory diseases, improve dental health, increase blood circulation, and much more. A single ounce of sesame seeds contains one-hundred and sixty calories, thirteen grams of healthy fats, five grams of protein, and three net carbs.

Flaxseeds are commonly used in low-carb baking. After all, a single ounce only contains half of a net carb while also having five grams of protein and eleven grams of heart-healthy fat. But these seeds have more benefits than their low-carb proprieties. Flaxseeds are full of omega-3 fatty acids, fiber, potassium, magnesium, calcium, iron, phosphorous, and certain B vitamins as well.

Flaxseeds are full of lignans, a plant compound and antioxidant which has been shown to greatly reduce the risk of both breast cancer and prostate cancer. In fact, flaxseeds contain up to eight-hundred times more lignans than other plants. One study of over six-thousand women found that those who regularly eat flaxseeds are eighteen percent less likely to develop breast cancer. Along with their anti-cancer benefits, these seeds also lower cholesterol, lower high cholesterol, and manage blood sugar.

Chapter 5:
Keto Vegetable Products

There is a reason that parents have long told children to eat their broccoli. Whether this cruciferous vegetable is eaten steamed or raw, it has many health benefits. In fact, some people even label broccoli as a 'superfood' due to it being an amazing source of vitamins - A, E, C, K, B vitamins, iron, calcium, selenium potassium, and fiber.

One of these vitamins, vitamin K, is essential for the natural clotting process in our blood as well as bone health and strength. Studies have even shown that if we increase our consumption of vitamin K, we may prevent osteoporosis and fractures as we age. We can easily consume more than our recommended intake with a single serving of broccoli. This makes broccoli a wonderful addition to your daily diet.

Broccoli: As if those weren't all good reasons to include broccoli on the Ketogenic diet, a single cup of this vegetable is only four net carbs. Whether you eat broccoli with Ranch dressing, cheese sauce, butter, bacon, or on its own, you are sure to find a way you can fully enjoy this vegetable ripe with benefits.

Kale and Spinach: Eating dark leafy greens is important, we all know that. Therefore, kale and spinach are so very popular. Kale and spinach taste different, but what about the nutritional differences? Firstly, both vegetables are full of vitamins and minerals. They have been shown to improve our cardiovascular health, immune system, bone health, and prevention of diseases as we age. The high content of vitamin C within these vegetables can even help our skin to age better.

Out of both vegetables, kale is higher in calories and carbohydrates. One hundred grams of kale contains forty-nine calories and five net carbohydrates whereas the same amount of spinach contains twenty-three calories and one net carb. That is quite a difference in carbohydrates. But kale is also higher in calcium and both vitamins K and A.

Mushroom: Mushrooms are commonly known as a superfood. This is because half of all edible mushrooms can benefit our health more than on just a basic nutritional need. They are known as a functional food because they can directly prevent and treat illnesses and disease. This has been shown to be true in both scientific studies and in practice for thousands of years in ancient Chinese medicine. This fungus contains antiviral, antibacterial, and ironically antifungal properties. They have also been shown to treat and reduce the risk of cancer, manage blood pressure, lower inflammation, strengthen the immune system, improve hair and skin health, lower cholesterol, and more.

Mushrooms are a tasty addition to the Ketogenic diet and incredibly low in carbohydrates. One-hundred ounces of white button mushrooms only contains two net carbohydrates.

Asparagus: Asparagus may be a popular vegetable, but did you know that it is part of the lily family? These little spears have many benefits, which are especially wonderful since one-hundred grams only contains about two net carbs. Asparagus is high in vitamins K, A, C, E, and B9 as well as phosphorous, fiber, potassium, and antioxidants. Studies have shown that this vegetable can improve your digestive health, nutrient absorption, cholesterol levels, manage blood pressure, and support a healthy pregnancy. Whether you are enjoying green, white, or purple asparagus, you will receive many benefits.

Bell Peppers: Bell peppers may be higher in carbs per gram than some options, but when enjoyed in moderation they are low enough to be fully enjoyed on the Ketogenic diet. This is great because they are also high in many nutrients. You can find one of the richest sources of vitamin C in bell peppers, along with vitamins K, B6, B9, E, and vitamin A as well as potassium. One bell pepper, or forty-five grams, contains four net carbs. This nightshade can help to reduce the risk of heart disease and cancer, boost the immune system, increase eye health, slow down aging, increase cognitive health, and promote a healthy pregnancy.

Green Beans: While beans are not usually allowed on the Ketogenic diet, green beans are the exception. These are young pole or bush beans that are extremely high in fiber and low in carbohydrates. In fact, while one-hundred grams of pinto beans contains forty-seven net carbohydrates, the same amount of green beans only contains four. They serve as wonderful sources for vitamin C, A, B6, K, fiber, calcium, iron, manganese, copper, potassium, and folic acid as well. The antioxidants within these beans have been shown to improve heart health and reduce the risk of developing heart disease. They also reduce the risk of colon cancer, boost the immune system, manage diabetes, strengthen bone health, improve eye health, treat gastrointestinal disorders, and improve pregnancy health.

Zucchini: The possibilities of cooking with zucchini are nearly limitless. One of many people's favorite ways to use this summer squash on the Ketogenic diet is to put it through a spiralizer and turn it into "noodles." These noodles can be made into a long list of pasta dishes at a fraction of the calorie and carb count. Actually, one-hundred grams of zucchini only contains two net carbs. This vegetable can also manage blood sugar, improve digestion, increase eye health, slow down aging, increase heart health, improve adrenal and thyroid functioning, lower inflammation, and boost energy levels.

Spaghetti Squash: Like zucchini, spaghetti squash can easily be made into low-carb pasta dishes. In fact, many people will roast and then stuff spaghetti squash with their favorite pasta toppings creating a decadent meal. One-hundred grams of this winter squash contains six net carbs. They are high in fiber and vitamins A, C, K, B9, as well as manganese. They are known to boost the immune system, reduce inflammation, increase lung health, manage blood circulation, strengthen bones, and much more.

Chapter 6:
Keto Fruits, Dairy, and Oil Products

Most fruits are high in glucose and fructose, causing a blood sugar spike and insulin response. Most are simply too high to be included on the Ketogenic diet. But that doesn't mean you have to forsake all fruits. Berries are an incredibly healthy source of fiber, vitamins, minerals, and antioxidants, all while being low enough in carbs to enjoy on the Ketogenic diet.

Strawberry: Strawberries are known to be a great source of vitamin C, vitamin B9 (folate), potassium, manganese, and antioxidants. This has been shown to improve the immune system, regulate blood sugar, lowers the risk of vision defects/cataracts, protect against cancer, treat arthritis, manage mood, lower allergic reaction severity, and more. One-hundred grams of strawberries contains six net carbohydrates.

Blueberry: Blueberries are higher in carbohydrates than strawberries, and therefore you are more limited in how many you can enjoy. Yet, they have many health benefits and are another good addition to the Ketogenic diet. This little berry is particularly high in fiber, manganese, vitamin C, vitamin K, and antioxidants. They are known to reduce cellular damage to our DNA, manage blood pressure, improve brain health and memory, reduce muscle damage, prevent heart disease, and more. These berries contain twice the number of net carbs as strawberries, with fifty grams containing six net carbs.

Olive: There are many benefits to eating olives, whether in their natural form or in the form of extra virgin olive oil. Many people may think that they are a vegetable, but they are in fact a fruit. While some have vaguely heard that olive oil is healthy, most haven't taken the time to learn its many health benefits. Worse yet, most people on the standard American diet eat a large portion of trans fats and fats with no nutritional properties rather than the amazing fats found in olives. Yet, this fruit has been shown to be high in antioxidants that protect against cancer, improve digestion, increase blood circulation, reduce inflammation, lower allergic reactions, increase brain function, reverse bone loss, manage blood pressure, and protect against infections.

This fruit is also high in essential omega-3 fatty acids, iron copper, sodium, calcium, and vitamin E. If you are interested in adding whole olives to your diet in addition to olive oil, you will be happy to know that a one-hundred-gram serving only contains three net carbs with ten grams of health-promoting fats.

Avocado: Avocados are one of the Ketogenic power foods. Sure, you can fully enjoy the Keto diet without avocados. But, the healthy fat, nutrient-dense, and low-carb fruit is the ideal of the Keto pyramid. One-hundred grams of this fruit, about half of a Haas avocado, only contains two net carbs. When eating avocados, you will be getting plenty of potassium, fiber, antioxidants, healthy fats, and vitamins K, B9, B5, B6, and E. In fact, while some people may be worried that bananas are non-Ketogenic and what that will mean for their potassium levels, avocados are much higher in potassium than a banana.

Dairy Products: Make use of dairy products such as yogurt, sour cream, cottage cheese, goat cheese, and whole milk.

I am a big fan of lard and olive oil (extra virgin) as they cook well and make food taste fantastic. Lard is good for the body. There are 12 grams of fat per serving, but only 5 grams of saturated fat. About half the fat in lard is Monounsaturated - you know the kind of fat that supposedly makes olive oil good for us. The saturated fat, of course, will primarily raise your HDL levels and that is a good thing if you ask me. The fatty-acid profile of lard is very similar to human body fat. And if you lose weight and consume your own fat in the process, that's good for you.

Butter is great, added salt or unsalted is fine. Stay away from fake butters such as margarine and vegetable oil butters, except if it is olive oil butter, however it must be 100% olive oil not 40 percent and the rest vegetable oil. I tell you to stay away from make believe butter not because they contain carbs but because of that pesky trans-fat (hydrogenated oils) that have been getting talked about lately. They are seriously not good for you and should not be included in anyone's diet. Extra-virgin olive oil is unrefined, low in fats and contains lots of antioxidants.

When it comes to the fat on the meat please do not remove the valuable fat off like a surgeon, not only will the food taste bland but you're missing out on precious fats' ability to help you burn up stored body fat. So, keep the steak fat on, the chicken skin, and bacon strips fat also. Remember we're not following the low-fat dogma high carbohydrate diet anymore.

Coconut oil boosts metabolism and ketosis. Grass-fed butter and ghee have lots of nutrients, antibiotics and good for use when on Keto diet. You may also use sesame oil and avocado oil.

Chapter 7:
Well Formulated Ketogenic Meals

Breakfasts

- Pancakes, made with eggs and cream cheese (add a little almond flour if you don't like the texture)

- Eggs

- Bacon

- Sausage

- Check the ingredients and avoid any added fillers such as rusk.

- Be careful of the ingredients in vegetarian sausages. Avoid those that have a high grain and sugar content. Don't worry about the salt at this stage – you need it!

- Mushrooms

- Tomatoes

- Cloud Bread (see the recipe in chapter 7)

Lunch

- Use cream cheese pancakes to roll sandwich ingredients inside, such as ham, cheese, egg, and mayo

- Salads with ingredients such as, lettuce, cucumber, bell peppers, radish, tomatoes

- You can add ingredients such as, tuna, cheese, or eggs to your salads

- Sprinkle seeds on your salad to add a crunchy texture

Dinner Meats

- Chicken drumsticks
- Chicken breast with soy sauce and sesame seeds
- Fish, such as salmon or cod
- Pork chops
- Ground beef
- Beef steaks

Dinner Vegetables

- Cauliflower
- Green leafy vegetables like bok choy, spinach, or chard

Dinner Sauces

- Add extra shredded cheese to cream cheese, then melt together to make a rich sauce

- Use Worcestershire, soy sauce, or mustard to add flavor to your sauces and gravies

Snacks

- Beef or chicken broth

- Avocado

- Around 10 nuts

- Unprocessed string cheese

Drinks

- Coffee with full-fat cream

- Green tea

- Water with lemon slices

- If you sweeten your drinks, use an alternative natural sweetener such as Stevia or Erythritol

- Red wine in the recommended moderation - you will need to deduct this from your carb count for the day

Chapter 8:
Finding Your Carb Sweet Spot

Most people consider a macronutrient breakdown of fat at 62%, protein at 28% while carbs stand at 10%. You can always cut down on carbs and protein to ensure that you burn more fat.

There are reasons why you need to trim down on protein. If you eat excess protein, the body converts it to glucose. In return, the level of blood insulin will rise, making the body to not get rid and burn the fat.

When it comes to the amount of carbs, do not cut the carb levels immediately with the intention of attaining your weight loss sweet spot. You can change to something closer to 30 to 50g net carbs each day and have a spike of 100 – 130g net carbs once or two times in a given week. This can be an awesome formula to ensure that you are in line with your weight loss goals. But if you aim at losing 20 to 25 pounds, you need to eat less than 20g of net carbs in a day.

You can aim at daily ration of 75% fat, 20% protein and 5% carbs. To get your sweet spot, include such items like leaf and fat lard, ghee, unprocessed beef tallow and coconut oil. Enjoy the grass-fed types of meat.

Do not cut on carbs drastically. Reduce the count slowly like around 40 to 50g until you attain your sweet spot.

Chapter 9:
Intermittent Fasting

In today's modern food culture, we have been conditioned for the entirety of our lives that we need to eat throughout the day to keep our bodies healthy. It commonly known that breakfast is a vital meal to kickstart the day, or that eating small meals every 2-3 hours is ideal for an efficient metabolism. The truth is, eating with this kind of frequency is not the way our species were made to function, and is a relatively new trend amongst humans.

By giving the body a break, such as following the intermittent fasting lifestyle, we can become a healthier, more efficient physical machine that performs at the level it was designed for. So, what is Intermittent Fasting? Answering this question is probably a good idea before we discuss any further details about it. Intermittent Fasting, put simply, is a diet protocol in which you do not eat throughout the day, only consuming all your daily calories within a specific eating window that you designate. The time that you spend fasting throughout the day is usually far longer than the eating window.

The key aspect to point out here is that you are not consuming any CALORIES during the fasting period, you are still free to consume as much water as you need (very important), as well as any flavored drinks or dietary supplements that you choose as long as they are calorie free. For example, most people that adhere to intermittent fasting engage in a 16-hour fast day, followed by an 8-hour eating window. One of the benefits of this protocol is that you can decide on your eating window based on your lifestyle, making intermittent fasting very convenient.

If you are an early bird, being most productive early in the day and usually in bed when the sun goes down, you can choose to eat earlier, say from 9am-5pm. For all the night owls out there, who see midnight on a regular basis, pushing you're eating window back to 4pm-12am is not a problem at all. Any way you design your intermittent fasting plan is fine, so long as you follow the foundational rules: no calories during your fasting period (while still staying properly hydrated) and sticking to consuming all your calories during the strict eating window that you designate.

If you are hearing intermittent fasting for the first time, you may be ready to close it immediately and never even consider this lifestyle. If that is you, this feeling is probably due to outdated fitness and nutrition advice that society and so-called "gurus" have hammered into your mind for decades. You have without a doubt heard that breakfast is the most important meal of the day, or eating 5-6 small meals every 2-3 hours throughout the day is the most effective way for efficient metabolism, or that 'starving' yourself to lose weight is counterproductive, etc.

Before we even begin to debunk these myths with all the benefits of intermittent fasting, you need to realize that this is not a new concept by any means. Eating throughout the course of the entire day is a relatively new concept. Food has become so convenient and accessible today that we are trained into believing we need three square meals a day. Society is so concerned with eating, instant gratification of our dietary desires that there are fast food restaurants on every corner with their flashing neon signs advertising the latest $5 calorie bomb. Is it any surprise then, that obesity levels are soaring, heart disease and stroke are running rampant, and people are unhealthier than ever before?

From our earliest ancestors all the way up until a few hundred years ago, the habit of eating one large meal at the end the day was the norm. Ancient humans were hunter-gatherers, spending the entire day foraging for edible vegetation, hunting game, and just trying to survive. Eating was considered a celebratory ritual and was accompanied by a feast each evening when the food was brought back to the tribe. Even our modern ancestors spent their days farming the land, working whatever job needed to be done for their families, eating one large meal after a hard day's work.

While I am by no means saying that these people had it better than we do now (I would rather eat a few too many calories each day than have to survive a saber-toothed tiger attack), they did in fact reap many of the benefits of intermittent fasting without even realizing it. To digress, eating throughout the duration of the day is a relatively new concept that is not at all necessary to a healthy lifestyle.

So, what exactly is intermittent fasting and why does it work? Intermittent Fasting (IF) may just be the best-kept secret of the diet and fitness industry. With over 100 years of research to back up this amazing game changing lifestyle, intermittent fasting is poised to take the health and wellness community by storm.

Before we jump into what intermittent fasting is, and why it works, let's first go over a couple of things that intermittent fasting is not.

First, intermittent fasting is NOT a diet plan. There are no off-limits foods, no meal plans, no meal prepping, and no complicated recipes. In fact, you can practice intermittent fasting and eat whatever you want. You'll still get some of the benefits. Of course, intermittent fasting works best when you try to eat more vegetables and whole foods, while eating less processed foods. It isn't necessary, and you can keep having treats without any guilt.

Second, intermittent fasting is NOT a metabolism lowering calorie restriction game. In fact, intermittent fasting can be used to lose weight, maintain weight, or even gain muscle. What does this mean for you? If you like intermittent fasting, and it ends up being a good fit, you can practice it for the rest of your life. It helps you lose weight, of course, but it has so many more benefits than just that.

Intermittent Fasting: The Basics

Let's get down to it. What is intermittent fasting? In short, intermittent fasting is a pattern of eating that involves periods of fasting, and periods of feasting. If this sounds frightening, don't worry! You've already been practicing the traditional eating pattern for your whole life.

This is what you've probably been taught: breakfast is the most important meal of the day, and you need to eat it about 30 minutes to 1-hour after you wake up. Your day should consist of three large meals, and two snacks. Many individuals have been made to believe this eating pattern is the best for our health.

But what if there was a body of research out there that proved otherwise? What if I told you that by not eating for periods of 16, 24, or even 36 hours, you could lose weight, gain muscle, and boost your energy levels and overall health? Well this is all true, and it's called intermittent fasting.

There are several different methods of intermittent fasting, and you will learn how to incorporate the top four in a later chapter. For now, let's just go over the basics. To practice intermittent fasting, you don't eat for 16+ hours. For most people, that means eating dinner at

7pm, going to sleep, and then not eating again until lunch the next day. Not eating for 16 hours might sound hard, but it becomes a lot easier if you sleep through 8 of those hours!

You may already have practiced intermittent fasting without realizing it. Have you ever woken up late on the weekend, or met a friend for a late brunch around noon? If that is your first meal of the day, you're practicing intermittent fasting.

If your first reaction to this is reluctance, keep reading. Over the next chapters, we will discuss why intermittent fasting is the right lifestyle for you and how you can easily integrate it into your life.

However, you may think to yourself, I'll be so hungry if I skip breakfast! We'll get more into this later, but after the first week or two, you really won't feel hungry! Your mind is used to eating in the morning, so for the first week, you will feel hungry. Once your brain learns to wait until lunch for food that hunger will go away. In many ways, intermittent fasting teaches you to listen to your body more closely.

The Science Behind the Lifestyle

To convince ourselves that intermittent fasting really is the lifestyle choice for us, let's go over a few of the scientific reasons why intermittent fasting causes weight loss without damaging our metabolism.

It is important to understand how chemistry that is external to our bodies has an impact on our fat loss and storage. Because when we say we want to lose weight, we mean that we want to lose fat. Now, most people follow the "calories in, calories out" method of weight loss. When you ingest fewer calories as compared to what you burn, you will lose weight. While this is true, researchers have now shown us that it leaves our metabolisms low, and we are almost guaranteed to put the weight back on.

Intermittent Fasting works because it doesn't rely on the calories in, calories out equation to promote weight loss. Instead, intermittent fasting prompts fat loss by lowering our insulin levels. So, how does insulin work?

Intermittent Fasting and Your Body's Chemistry
Insulin tells our body when it is time to store energy as fat, and when it is time to burn fat as energy. When we eat, our stomach and liver turn food into energy. Some of that energy goes into our blood stream as blood sugar, and we use that immediately. The rest? Stored as fat.

Insulin is a chemical, released by our pancreas when we eat, that tells our body it is time to store fat. So, when we don't eat for 16 hours or more, our insulin level goes down significantly, and our body transitions into the fat burning mode. So, even if you ate a large dinner the night before, you'll still go into fat burning mode the next morning!

Insulin isn't the only chemical that a fast trigger, however. When we fast for longer than 16 hours, our body produces more human growth hormone (HGH). This fantastic hormone tells our body to burn fat, repair muscle, and even build new muscles! By fasting, you will lose weight and have more energy!

Yet there is even one more reason that intermittent fasting kicks the calories in calories out method of weight loss: when you fast for over 16 hours, your body produces more adrenaline. Adrenaline, in turn, gives you more energy and mental awareness! You'll feel energetic and thoughtful even when you haven't eaten recently.

The combination of these three effects, lower insulin, increased HGH, and increased adrenaline, combine in your body to raise your metabolism, sometimes up to 14% higher than your base rate. This boost in metabolism can lead to some great weight loss results! You will also be reducing your calories somewhat, since you eat fewer meals each day. This slight calorie reduction, plus increased metabolism, will lead to fantastic and long-lasting results.

How IF Works

For you to understand how intermittent fasting works, it is important to understand how the body processes the food you eat.

When you eat (if you follow the USDA's food pyramid, which entails high carb, minimal fat and moderate protein intake), the body goes into a fed state i.e. a state in which the body has high levels of various nutrients in the bloodstream. The fed state lasts for about 3-5 hours after which your body goes into a post-absorptive state where nothing is being digested although the levels of insulin are still high in the blood. This is the time the cells are taking up any remaining blood glucose for use or storage. During this period (the fed state and post absorptive state, the body is actively digesting everything you've eaten so that some can be absorbed into the bloodstream for transportation to different parts of the body where the cells in various parts use them for energy.

After the food is absorbed and is in the bloodstream for transportation to different parts of the body, one challenge arises though; the cells don't have their own mechanism for absorbing glucose from the bloodstream. In fact, they can only do that with the aid of insulin, a hormone secreted by the pancreas in response to rising blood glucose concentrations. The purpose of insulin is simple; to 'open the gates' to the cells so that they can take up the glucose in the bloodstream in order to maintain a healthy level of blood glucose concentration. This essentially means that even if there is an excess of blood glucose (after the fed state), the presence of insulin in the bloodstream keeps the 'doors' open so that the cells take up more glucose. They don't use everything though; the excess glucose is first converted into glycogen, which is then stored in the liver.

Glycogen is like an emergency/backup source of energy, which kicks in when glucose levels in the blood are low for an extended period. But the glycogen stores are limited; they can only take about 2000kcal of energy at any given time. So, if there is still an excess of glucose available for the cells, it is converted into fatty acids and glycerol, which are then stored in the various fat stores around the body e.g. around organs, under the skin etc. The thing is; the presence of insulin in the bloodstream tends to promote fat storage and inhibits fat burning.

The entire process i.e. being in the fed state (up to the time the body no longer has any glucose which needs to be used up in the bloodstream) takes about 10-12 hours after you've had your meal. If you don't take any more food, this is when you start entering the fasted state, a state where the body has no more glucose in the bloodstream but is 'hungry' for nutrients. What does it do? Well, it goes to its backup power source i.e. glycogen, which it converts into glucose for use in different body processes with the help of glucagon (another hormone secreted by the pancreas) in the liver. At this time, the body doesn't just break down glycogen exclusively; it starts loosening up its grip on other energy stores e.g. the fat stores so that they can be burned to fuel different body processes. This means when you are in a fasted state (i.e. after 12-14 hours from your last meal), you can be sure of losing weight without struggle. The goal of intermittent fasting is to induce the fasted state by spacing meals in a manner that you get to a fasted state every single day so as to push your body to the point of starting to burn glycogen (and perhaps deplete it a little) so that it can start burning more stored fat for energy.

The challenge with most of us is that we hardly get to the fasted state; we are very used to eating breakfast, lunch and dinner in some predetermined structure. The challenge though is that this 'structure' hardly gets us into a fasted state. In fact, we are always in the fed state, as many of us eat many meals about 4-5 hours apart. Obviously, this results in a nutrient overload and always keeps us in the fed state because this essentially keeps the body in the fed state. It is only after dinner when we try to get to the fasted state while we are asleep. But given that many of us take breakfast quite early and delay our dinner time, we hardly really 'get there.'

Do you know that this has great adverse effects on your body? Well, let me explain.

As you already know, most of the time, our bodies are in the fed state and not the fasted state making our cells more adapted to burning glucose instead of fat for energy. This simply means that normally, the levels of insulin are always high. There is a problem though; with insulin levels always high, the cells start becoming more 'blind' to the signals of insulin such that more insulin is required to trigger the cells to open to take up glucose. This is referred to as insulin resistance. In such a state, the body is always burning glucose and rarely ever burns fat (the presence of insulin has fat burning inhibitory properties) and when the glucose is depleted, the body doesn't move to the fasted stage; instead, it gets hungry for more glucose. This is because the body has less capacity to mobilize and burn fat for energy. So, you can picture the cravings and the excess fat storage that comes with insulin resistance.

The secret to weight loss is in structuring your meals in a manner that ensures you get your 12-14 hours minimum from the time you had your last meal to the next. The rest of the hours i.e. 12-10 hours are up to you; eat whatever you want but just don't overindulge! With fasting, this process goes on reverse. When you don't eat for an extended period, the levels of insulin fall as a result of falling blood glucose levels, which signals the body to burn stored energy (glycogen and fats) since no more is coming in. This brings about weight loss in the long term.

From the above explanation, the period within which you stay without food ought to start from about 12-14 hours (no less). If you want to fast for longer, you are free to do that; this brings about fasted effects because you get to use more of the stored fats for energy. The feeding window therefore is within 10-8 hours or less (not more).

Note: You can increase the fasting hours to achieve greater benefits. To simplify things, you can follow different intermittent fasting protocols, which we will discuss later.

So how exactly does intermittent fasting result to weight loss? Well, there are different explanations to this.

- You effectively create a calorie deficit when you fast.

Powerful Ketogenic Diet and Intermittent Fasting Secrets

- You ultimately are likely to consume fewer calories within the feeding window, something which will create the much-needed calorie deficit for weight loss

- You enhance your metabolism with intermittent fasting.

Chapter 10:
Why Try Intermittent Fasting

By following this protocol, you are far more likely to consume fewer calories during the day. The foundation of any weight loss plan is often lost behind complicated diet plans and flawed philosophies that serve to confuse people more than they help them. This foundation is that calories are the key to weight gain or loss. If you consume fewer calories per day than your body burns, you are going to lose weight. Likewise, if you take in a surplus of calories compared to what your body burns, weight gain is inevitable.

What happens when we eat regular meals all throughout the day? You wake up, eat breakfast, and then usually even before lunch you get hungry again, indulging in a snack here and there. After lunch, we usually have a 4-6-hour wait before dinner and then more snacks to satisfy our urges tend to follow. With this constant cycle of eating, getting full, and then getting hungry again and eating more between meals, it makes it so easy for us to consume too many calories throughout the day. With intermittent fasting, once your body adjusts to the prolonged fasting period, you will eat fewer meals because you are limited to a timed 'feeding' window. This allows you to prevent excess hunger between meals and feel relatively satiated throughout the duration.

For example, the average person is advised to follow a 2,000-calorie per day diet. Which one is challenging to achieve, eating throughout the entire day, 3 meals and snacks included, while only consuming 2,000 calories, or only allowing yourself 8 hours to eat the same number? Obviously, it is easier to eat a healthy number of calories if you limit them to a shorter window. Intermittent fasting will allow you to more easily consume your desired number of calories than eating all day will.

Another profound benefit of intermittent fasting is an increase in insulin sensitivity in the body. As we discussed earlier, our society is experiencing an obesity epidemic of epic proportions. Hand in hand with obesity is type 2 diabetes. Type 2 diabetes results when the body is unable to use insulin properly. When this happens, the pancreas (the organ that produces insulin) will attempt to produce extra insulin at first, but will eventually be unable to keep up, causing blood glucose levels to soar.

Obesity is associated with type 2 diabetes due to the fact that when the pancreas has to constantly release a large amount of insulin (typical of a poor diet, a primary cause of obesity), eventually the insulin receptors in the body become overloaded and lose their ability to use insulin efficiently. Almost 90% of the people living with type 2 diabetes are obese or overweight.

As we discuss obesity, losing weight, and burning fat, let's use basic human biology to explain why we store fat in the first place. The human body is an incredible machine, it is designed to survive many hardships, and famine is one of them. When we consume an excess of calories, the body will use as many calories as it needs at the time, but then stores away the rest as either glycogen in the liver, but more readily, as adipose tissue (or fat).

This was extremely necessary for the ancient man, when food was scarce and unavailable for sometimes days on end; the body used the fat it had stored during times of plentiful food to survive. Fat, however, is not the body's go to source for fuel in normal situations. If food is readily available, it will use glucose as a primary energy source, saving the fat for more drastic times. In today's world, with eating all throughout the day is the norm and food more readily available than ever before, the average person's body today tends to get its energy almost exclusively from glucose. We never experience that famine situation in which our fat stores were designed to withstand.

As advanced as we think we've become in our society, it is ironic that our actual genome has changed very little since ancient humans. Even today, if we engage in intermittent fasting, we signal to the body that we are experiencing a period of scarce food and, once the body gets used to this protocol, we see a shift in its primary energy source. By following the intermittent fasting protocol, we can train the body to start using our fat stores for energy instead of glucose alone. Most overweight people today are caught in a cycle where the blood glucose is always elevated due to being full. When this starts to decrease, instead of their body switching to burning fat as fuel, they simply get hungry and eat again. This not only keeps blood glucose way too high consistently, but also does not allow the body to burn fat like it otherwise would.

Another little known but monumental benefit of intermittent fasting is that it has been shown to decrease the odds of contracting breast cancer in women, and aid in the fight against cancer in general once a woman has developed it. A study of 7,000 women with a history of anorexia showed a 50% reduction in the incidence of breast cancer. Before we go any further yes, anorexia is a horrible disease but what researchers took from this was that caloric restriction and fasting, all characteristic of anorexia, decreases breast cancer risks. Intermittent fasting reduces the side effects of chemotherapy and even increase its effectiveness when used immediately before and after chemo.

What an enormous benefit to gain from a change in diet. Literally everything we do with proper nutrition and exercise, goes back to trying to live if we can and be healthy while we are here. Intermittent fasting has consistently shown to increase the lifespan of numerous animals, which is what you and I are as well! Not to mention that living a healthy and happy life is one of the most important things to do while we live on this beautiful planet.

Another positive side effect associated with intermittent fasting is improved brain health. We can agree that the brain is an important organ to look out for, as even agreeing with this statement requires the brain. Prolonged periods of fasting slowed down the flow of information across the neurons in the brain. Although slowing down our brains may seem counter intuitive, this benefits our mental health.

The stress of day-to-day life which we all experience has our neuronal circuits constantly firing, leaving the brain overworked by our tedious schedules. Too much activity in the synapses of the brain, (which are responsible for relaying information) has been linked with several diseases of the brain and nervous system, such as Alzheimer's and Parkinson's disease. It seems as if the slowing down of the brain through fasting gives it a break, allowing it to recharge. When in a fasting state, the body produces compounds known as ketone bodies, which are known to protect the neurons in the brain, preventing them from degrading to the point of disease. Furthermore, intermittent fasting has even been proven extremely effective in combating depression and anxiety.

'Brain-derived neurotrophic factor' is a chemical released in the brain that is responsible for the formation of neuronal networks. In people suffering from depression, we see this chemical suppressed substantially. When these new neuronal networks have a difficult time forming and branching out, depression is far more likely. A study from the Neurobiology of Disease in 2007 concluded that periods of fasting can increase the concentration of Brain-Derived Neurotrophic factor anywhere from 50 to 400 percent! We're not talking about a slight increase here; this is a huge amount.

Another chemical chain that occurs in the brain during periods of fasting and caloric restriction, involves a hormone called Ghrelin. Ghrelin is known as the hunger hormone because it increases when we are hungry and/or fasting. When it comes to mental health, however, increased Ghrelin is very helpful. Not only has this hormone been linked to elevated mood, it is a natural antidepressant and promotes neurogenesis in the brain.

In our world today, chronic depression and anxiety levels are at an all-time high, and people report feeling higher levels of anxiety than ever before. Intermittent fasting is a good consideration to circumvent this trend and help keep your mood uplifted throughout the day. Not only will this lifestyle alter the chemical balance in your brain, allowing you to combat and prevent depression, but the weight-loss and fitness benefits will serve to improve your self-image and confidence, which are both aspects of life that, when negative, cause depression and anxiety. Think of intermittent fasting as a double-edged sword that slices through both obesity and depression.

Intermittent fasting may seem to be a new trend that has emerged in the spotlight recently, as many fad diet plans often do, but rest assured that this is not a recent new way of life. This lifestyle has been around far longer than you and I have been alive, or even our great-great (times 20) grandparents have been around to consider it.

Today's modern food culture has led us to believe that we must not go any more than a few hours without eating, and that our entire day should be based around meals. The science behind intermittent fasting does not agree. Should you choose to give this lifestyle a try, you could reap all the benefits that we've discussed and more. While skipping meals and engaging in a prolonged period of fasting may go against all your prior beliefs on eating and how food should be consumed, I strongly believe that you will find the benefits worth the try.

More About Weight Loss

Your body tends to store energy in the form of fat cells. When you don't eat anything, there a couple of different changes that take place in your body that help your body access its energy reserves, and in the activity of your nervous system. Here are what takes place in the metabolism of your body whenever you fast.

Insulin- The level of insulin increases whenever you eat. So, while you are fasting, the insulin levels in your body will decrease. A low level of insulin means that it is easier for your body to burn the fats that are stored within.

Human Growth Hormone - The human growth hormone or HGH level increases when you fast. This hormone is responsible for not just fat loss, but it also helps with muscle gain and it kick starts autophagy.

Noradrenaline - Norepinephrine or noradrenaline is sent to the fat cells by the nervous system to help break down the fat in the body and to free up the reserves of fatty acids to provide energy.

If you keep consuming food throughout the day, then it is unlikely that any of these changes will take place. Short-term fasting helps increase your body's ability to burn fats. So, a short-term fast like intermittent fasting induces several changes in your body that makes it easier to burn fat. It also reduces the production of insulin while increasing the production of the growth hormone and epinephrine to give a metabolic boost to your body.

Intermittent fasting helps you reduce your intake of calories and helps with weight loss. The primary reason why intermittent fasting is an effective weight loss technique is because it reduces your calorie intake. As such there is no calorie restrictions prescribed by this diet. All the different methods of intermittent fasting involve foregoing meals during the periods of fast. Unless you try to compensate for all this by eating more during the eating window, then you will certainly be consuming fewer calories than usual. Intermittent fasting can be a major contributor to weight loss if you carefully follow the protocols of this diet for at least three weeks. It isn't just fat loss that you will experience on this diet; you will also notice that you are losing fat from your abdominal region. The benefits of intermittent fasting are not restricted to just weight loss. This diet has a positive effect on your metabolic health and helps prevent any chronic diseases.

You don't have to necessarily count calories while following any method of intermittent fasting, but you need to maintain a calorie deficit if you want to lose weight. Intermittent fasting helps reduce your calorie intake without setting up any calorie restrictions.

One of the side effects of a diet that helps you lose fat is that it also causes you to burn muscle while burning fat. When it comes to intermittent fasting, you will not be burning any muscle mass and, in fact, it helps you gain lean muscle mass. The reduction in muscle mass while on intermittent fasting is quite low when compared to a diet that prescribes continuous calorie restriction.

Apart from this, it is also easier to eat healthily while following this diet. The simplicity of this diet is the main reason for all the benefits it offers. You can select any method of intermittent fasting and you will notice that you are eating healthier meals than before. If you want to follow the OMAD protocol, then you can eat only one meal per day. If you can eat only one meal, then you need to make sure that the meal that you eat will fill you up so that you can go through the day without feeling hungry. The foods that will fill you up for longer are foods rich in protein and fiber. So, knowingly or not you will start to incorporate healthy foods into your diet. For instance, eating a bowl of lettuce will make you feel fuller for longer than a packet of chips. So, you will be making healthier food choices.

Intermittent fasting is a wonderful dieting protocol that you can follow to lose weight. The main reason for weight loss on this diet is the reduction in the intake of calories.

So, by now, you know all that you must know about Intermittent Fasting and if you are willing to try this great lifestyle, I would be glad to make your life easier. In this very short section, I am going to give you some tips that you can use so you can deal with hunger and stick to your plan.

When I first started intermittent fasting it was like one year ago, I found about it from one of the best trainers out there in my opinion and it was one of the best things that I did to implement this in my life. I was not eating in the morning anyway, so it was easier for me to get started, but what really helped me out were his little tricks about making it easier, almost effortless to keep. One of the best things that you can do is to start drinking coffee and I mean black coffee without any sugar or milk. Why do you want to do this? Because black coffee is a great appetite suppressor, it helps you manage your hunger and for sure if you want to have a sensation of fullness you may want to drink it with sparkling water as well.

Christine Moore

The last thing that I will mention is that it is easier to spend 4-8 hours after waking up without food. You can drink some cups of coffee with some water and this will help you manage your hunger much better.

Chapter 11:
Keto and Intermittent Fasting

Intermittent fasting and the Ketogenic diet are both hot topics that often fall into conversations these days, especially in the health and fitness industry. Some differences make you wonder if one is better than the other, or if they can both fit into your life.

Let's now compare intermittent fasting and the Ketogenic diet. We've already covered what each one does in the previous chapters, so let's see some brief similarities and differences that they share. Afterward, we will discuss some important tips on how to intermittent fast on the Ketogenic diet.

Similarities
Ketosis is a direct result of starving the body of either carbs or food in general. Therefore, the Ketogenic diet and intermittent fasting have much of the same benefits. They work with each other very well as they are aiming towards the same goal, entering and maintaining ketosis.

Just like the Ketogenic diet, intermittent fasting involves times of starving the body of either carbs or food. However, because you are still eating food on the Ketogenic diet, intermittent fasting gets the body into ketosis faster, because you're having no carbs or food at all when you're in the fasting state.

If you look at intermittent fasting and the Ketogenic diet, you can see that each one complements the other. Both have benefits for weight loss and health, and that has more to do with fasting than ketosis.

Differences

The most obvious and main difference is, one involves eating while the other doesn't. You can eat throughout the day and stay in ketosis when doing the Ketogenic diet. Whereas intermittent fasting means you won't eat any food for a certain amount of time.

The Ketogenic diet's goal is to put your body into ketosis. Intermittent fasting isn't a diet and just because you choose to do it, doesn't mean your goal is to be in ketosis. Some intermittent fast just to eat less during the day and to keep from overeating at night. Somebody might choose to do a Keto diet for more than just to lose weight.

Trying to Intermittent Fast on The Ketogenic Diet

- Don't try to intermittent fast in the first two weeks of starting the Ketogenic diet or if you follow the Standard American Diet. This is extremely important. Your body requires to get adapted to the Keto diet before you try intermittent fasting. Your body must get used to eating low carbs so your body can utilize ketones for energy instead of using glucose. If you try intermittent fasting at the same time you begin the Keto diet, you will not succeed. You will be too glucose-dependent and too hungry to stick with it. There is some misinformation around about intermittent fasting. Intermittent fasting needs to be natural and not a struggle, and you should never feel hungry. It will be a gradual process and take time before it is used effectively.

- Don't try to plan intermittent fasting too much. You must listen to your body. Intermittent fasting works best if it is done naturally. If you realize its lunchtime, but you don't feel hungry, just skip it and eat at dinner time. If it is too late to eat? Skip dinner and eat breakfast. Most individuals are at ease to skip breakfast anyway. Try to eat about 1 pm and eat again about four hours before you go to bed, so your body has time to digest your foods.

- Start slow. Don't force yourself to do the complete intermittent fasting schedule immediately. You should never deprive or restrict yourself. When your body has become fat-adapted, you won't feel as hungry. Begin by staying away from snacks between meals. Next, try skipping regular meals. Do this only if you don't feel hungry.

- Stay busy. You might find it easier to skip meals if you are busy and don't spend time in the kitchen. You might be tempted to have a snack if you are around food, even if you don't feel hungry. It is easy to go without food when you are out shopping. Remember to drink plenty of liquid. Water, tea, or coffee is all you need.

Intermittent fasting is just one tool to help you reach your goal. It helps with weight loss, longevity, and many other things, but it is just one factor that helps you meet your target. Exercise, micronutrients, macronutrients, enough sleep, and stress levels are some things to consider. Never use intermittent fasting as a quick fix when you have overindulged.

Butter or bulletproof coffee will break your fasting. Eating coconut oil or butter will not keep you in a fasted state. Anything that has calories will have the same effect. That's why it is called fasting. If you must have coffee in the mornings, add some cream but skip the sugar, butter, and oils.

Remember as I mentioned earlier, intermittent fasting isn't for everyone. If you come under any of the conditions below you should not do intermittent fasting:

- Type 1 diabetes

- Type 2 diabetics should only do it under a doctor's supervision since they might need to adjust their medication.

- Bulimia nervosa

- Anorexia nervosa
- Adrenal or chronic fatigue disorders
- Breastfeeding
- Pregnant women
- Very stressed
- Exercise too much
- Don't get enough sleep

If you experience any side effects such as hormone imbalance, irregular periods, anxiety, or sleeplessness, you should consult your health care practitioner before continuing.

Chapter 12:
Intermittent Fasting Regiments

You also need to understand everything you can about what intermittent fasting does to your body, your mind, and your life. When you understand the kind of lifestyle you are getting into and the benefits you stand to gain, then you will be able to persevere and eventually practice intermittent fasting happily and diligently. Some of the protocols you may want to look at include;

- Eat-stop-eat protocol
- The 16-8 protocol
- The 5:2 fast diet
- The alternate-day fasting
- One meal a day (OMAD)

16:8 Method
The 16:8 method (16 hours OFF and 8 hours ON) of Intermittent Fasting is the easiest and least hunger-inducing version of IF to integrate into

your life. It is also known as the daily window fasting. This method works on its own, or as a stepping-stone towards longer fasts.

To practice 16:8 IF, you simply fast for 16 hours in a day, then eat for an 8-hour window. This is the shortest fast and the longest feasting window of any of the forms of intermittent fasting. When you follow 16:8 fasting method, you eat within the 8-hour window (maybe, 11 a.m. – 7 p.m.) and then fast for the remaining 16 hours (7 p.m. until 11 a.m.). The fasting and eating window can vary depending on the individual.

Alternate Day Fasting

This fasting has several different versions. Some of them allow consumption of 500 calories during the fast to make things easy. Starting with a 24-hour fast may be difficult for a beginner like you. True fast lovers will enjoy fasting 24 hours once or twice a week.

Eat Stop Eat (24-Hour Fast)

With this method, you fast for 24-hours once or twice every week. To start fasting, you start the fast after Saturday night dinner and fast until Sunday night dinner. This will give you a full 24-hour fast. Also, you can try a breakfast to breakfast or lunch to lunch method. You can drink water, tea, coffee and other non-caloric beverages during the fast. To lose weight, you must eat a normal amount of food during your eating period. Meaning, you shouldn't try to compensate for your lost meals due to the fast. You can start with 16 hours fast and then gradually increase the time.

5:2 Diet

This diet is called the Fast Diet. The diet recommends that you eat as usual for 5 days of the week and then eat 500 to 600 calories (men 600 calories, women 500 calories) daily during the remaining 2 days.

The Warrior Diet (20/4)

The Warrior diet is a combination of exercise and fasting. You will need to follow your gut feeling when it comes to choosing the right diet. Avoid getting tempted by processed food or junk food. Don't get too rigid with the types of macronutrients and calories that need to be consumed during the eating window. Instead, as the name implies, eat like a warrior! Our prehistoric warriors had little food during the day and had their meal at night, i.e., little food in the day and more food at night. After 20 hours, you can eat whatever foods you want if it is within a four-hour eating window.

The Warrior diet is more to do with vigorous exercising (even during the fasting days) and controlled food-intake. You will need to exercise when your stomach is completely empty (preferably as soon as you wake up). You will have only one meal in a day. If you can adapt to this type of intermittent fasting, you will be able to burn more fat (into energy) and will get a lean physique without the need to count your calories.

Your exercise routine should be total body strength training – squats, pushups, pull-ups, high jumps, skipping and presses. You can also include high-intensity cardio exercises, such as frog jumps or sprints, in between these sessions. These sessions can last for between 20 and 45 minutes.

Make sure you have a healthy organic, wholesome meal during your eating window. Add more vegetables, spices, greens and fruit to your plate. Drink enough water after your meal.

One Meal a Day Diet

The popularity of intermittent fasting is increasing every day. One method of IF that is steadily becoming quite popular is the One Meal a Day diet also known as the OMAD diet. Abstaining from food helps modulate your body's performance and when you fast for prolonged periods, it has a positive effect on your body and mind.

The OMAD protocol is designed in such a manner that the fasting ratio you need to follow is 23:1. It means that your body will be effectively fasting for 23 hours and the eating window is restricted to one hour. If you want to burn fat, trigger weight loss, improve your mental clarity and reduce the time that you spend on food, then eating one meal a day is a brilliant idea.

The OMAD method oscillates between periods of eating and fasting. This method of fasting reduces the eating window more than the other diets. While following this dieting protocol, you need to make sure that you consume your daily calories within one meal, and you fast for the rest of the day. OMAD helps you reap all the benefits of intermittent fasting and it simplifies your schedule as well. The ideal time to break your fast is between 4 and 7 p.m. When you do this, you give your body enough time to start digesting the food that you eat before you sleep.

From the perspective of evolution, humans aren't designed to eat three meals per day. As mentioned earlier, our ancestors' bodies were used to functioning optimally even when there was food scarcity. Intermittent fasting protocols like the OMAD tend to kickstart various cell functions in your body that are helpful to improve your overall health. It can be a challenge starting out with this method of dieting. There are three simple tips that you can follow to make the transition easier on yourself.

The first thing that you need to do is slowly cut back on the carbs that you consume. If you want to optimize the results of this diet and want the least amount of crankiness, then you must limit your carb intake. Your body tends to create a stock of glycogen in the body when lots of carbs are taken in. If there is always some glucose present in your body, then your body will not be able to shift into ketosis. Ketosis is essential to kickstart the process of burning fats. So, if you are trying to start this diet, then it is a good idea to start by slowly cutting back on your carb intake.

You need to ease your body into getting used to this fasting protocol. It can be quite difficult to go from eating three meals a day to just one meal a day. You need to ease the transition so that it doesn't feel like you are suffering. A simple way in which you can do this is by slowly getting your body used to the idea of eating fewer meals. So, if you are used to eating three meals per day and tend to snack in between the meals, then the first step is to eliminate all the snacks. Then you make gradual increments to the time between the meals and cut down on the number of meals you eat. If you do this, it will be quite easy to follow this diet.

Another simple way in which you can make this diet easier on your body is to consume some caffeine. A morning cup of coffee (devoid of milk and sugar) will make you feel fuller for longer and will keep your hunger pangs at bay. You will learn more about the different tips that you can follow to manage your hunger in the coming chapters.

Chapter 13:
Beginners 4 Week Plan

To start the Keto lifestyle is simple; many health and fitness "experts" make the Keto diet complicated. Here are the key points to getting started the right way with the Keto diet.

- You can eat generous servings of any type of meat, don't trim the fat off.

- You can eat all the vegetables you wish, just watch the carb count on veggies such as broccoli.

- You can have salads with most dressings.

- You can eat most cheeses.

- Use mayonnaise and olive oil on everything.

- Keep deviled eggs ready for yourself as a snack.

- Get creative with your meal choices; if it's an omelet, make it a bacon, cheddar, diced tomato and mushroom omelet.

- Eat when you're hungry not by a schedule.
- Drink lots of water to get rid of impurities in the body and to stave off constipation.

If you have a craving and binge on ice cream or cookies, don't worry just go right back on the diet after that last meal. You can have all the coffee and tea you want if add-ons such as milk, sugar, syrup and the like don't take you over your set carb count. Stay away from most sugary foods for the first 6 days, such as honey, jelly, syrups, cake, rice, cereals. Sunday go all out on whatever you like.

A Word on Cheating

If you must have that bagel or bowl of rice during the first week, go for it; don't beat yourself up over it. I want you to feel freedom over food not feel like a victim. And the same goes for if you lost all the weight you wanted and fell off and ate the wrong foods, no big deal. When following the Keto diet, there are things that you should consider:

1. This diet is not for everyone. Those who are undergoing medical attention such as cardiovascular diseases, gallbladder, diabetes, and pregnant women are discouraged from following this diet.

2. The Ketogenic diet should not be combined with other diets. Doing so could only compromise your health. Therefore, choose which diet really works for you. Before starting with a new one, allow your body to rest and adjust for at least 2 weeks.

3. Consult with your nutritionist. Ask a nutritionist to supervise your progress even if you are at your fittest. If you are into strength training, it is more important to consult a nutritionist. This kind of diet requires careful meal planning as it is easy to slip and go back to your usual eating habit especially when you find the diet uncomfortable and maintaining it becomes a bit of a challenge.

4. Drink plenty of water. If there is one major drawback of the Keto diet, that would have to be constipation. Since water is flushed out from the body quickly, there is usually a delay in bowel movement. Therefore, drinking plenty of water along with consuming food rich in fiber is important while on the Ketogenic Diet.

You're ready to go shopping. It can be an overwhelming task at first, so here are some helpful tips to keep you on track. Plan your meals ahead before heading to the grocery or store. Write all your ingredients and know what you need and what you already have. Do your purchases on a seasonal basis and note when there is abundance of fresh produce? Some of the items to purchase:

- Keto meats – steaks, ground beef, shrimp, pork chops, bacon, salmon

- Keto vegetables – broccoli, kale, cucumber, asparagus, spinach, peppers, cauliflower, mushrooms, squash

- Keto fruits – almost all berries

- Dairy products – half and half, butter, most cheese like Parmesan, cream, Swiss, blue, shredded cheddar

- Other Keto pantry items – almonds, hazelnuts, cocoa powder, macadamia, sunflower seeds, olives, all the spices, coconut oil

Always buy the items in bulk. This is a wonderful way of saving money. Be ready to buy when there are offers or coupons before they expire.

Start with the Keto Diet First

By starting with the Keto Diet first, it will help you transition your body into a ketosis state, so you begin to burn excess fat for energy to facilitate weight loss. By consuming low glycemic fruits and leafy green vegetables, moderate high-quality protein and significant healthy fats will increase your satiety and help you feel full.

However, minimize and eliminate all processed foods wherever possible including sugar. While this may be difficult initially (I know as I was in the same place), you will see benefits much quicker. This sets up well to integrate Intermittent Fasting next with your Keto Diet as your body will be already accustomed to being in a fat burning state.

Integrate Intermittent Fasting Next

Intermittent Fasting promotes weight loss as well, improves your key physiology functions and detoxifies your body. You can amplify these benefits when you combine Intermittent Fasting with the Keto Diet.

Select your fasting protocol. The most popular method of Intermittent Fasting is a time restricted feeding (TRF) protocol as discussed earlier called 16/8. This means you don't eat for 16 hours and consume your meals within an eight (8) hour window. The 16/8 protocol will be the easiest to start with since it's close to what you normally do. You can then transition to longer periods of fasting as your body adjusts to fasting on a regular basis.

As you fast, your body reaches into its stores of glycogen to provide energy to your body. Once your glycogen stores are depleted, your body will begin to burn stored fat to provide energy once ketosis begins. Fasting assists the body to enter ketosis since there is no other source of energy available during the fasting period.

Break Your Fast with Keto-Friendly Wholesome Foods

The next step is to eat Keto-friendly foods when you break your fast. For instance, if you're eating window stretches from noon until 8 pm at night then the food that you can consume during this period must be Keto-friendly. Use the Keto food list to make sure that you always have Keto ingredients and supplies in your pantry. Go through the various recipes given in this book to cook tasty and healthy food.

You may also experiment a little before getting the perfect combination of the various Intermittent Fasting protocols, the Keto Diet and your personal lifestyle.

Always consult your physician before you start the Keto Diet and any of the Intermittent Fasting protocols.

The goal of the transitional phase on the Keto diet is to allow you to ease into your new lifestyle. While it is certainly possible to jump right into a new lifestyle, it is not the easiest or most encouraging approach. We are all struggling with enough difficulties in life already. There is no need to challenge yourself to do a one-eighty lifestyle shift when instead you can ease into confidently over the span of four weeks.

There's some stuff you need to do as preparation for the Keto Diet journey to come! It helps to have all your helpful tools assembled before you begin, so that you're fully prepped and ready to go. That includes purchasing a Keto Blood or Breath monitor, buying the necessary cooking implements and kitchen tools for making Keto meals, and investing in a new notebook as your food diary. You'll also want to go online and find a Macro calculator. Fill out the questionnaire and then write the results here:

- Fats: _____ grams
- Proteins: _____ grams

- Carbohydrates: _____ grams

- Total Calories: _____

It's also helpful to set goals. How much weight are you intending to lose by the end of these four weeks? Do you have any other Keto Diet goals? Add those to your food diary to help you stay on track.

- Weight Loss goal: _____ pounds in _____ weeks

- Fitness goal: _____

You may also want to come up with a meal plan for your first week. Include the recipes that you'll need, too. You'll also want to purchase the ingredients for at least the first seven days of Keto meals, based on your personalized Macros.

You'll notice in Week One there's no exercise plan (yet). That's because we want your body to get used to Intermittent Fasting before we add exercise to it. Let's just focus on your eating plan and eating schedule. There's plenty of time to add exercise later!

Whew! There's a lot to do before Day 1, but these are all the foundational tools you'll need to get through your first week, both Keto dieting and Intermittent Fasting. Now you're ready to start and you've laid the groundwork for a successful first month!

Week One

Powerful Ketogenic Diet and Intermittent Fasting Secrets

Day 1

Day 1 is going to be a normal, regular day without any major changes to your Ketogenic Diet at all. We're going to ease slowly into Intermittent Fasting. So, for today all you've got to do is cook and eat three regular Keto meals plus a snack/dessert/drink. Follow your own customized meal plan. You can also eat your meals whenever you want. Make sure you reach your Macros. Track what you ate in your food diary. Monitor either your breath or blood and check for ketosis.

There are no specific guidelines about exactly when you should measure ketone levels. In the morning, ketone concentrations are lower and higher in the evening. Two factors throw off ketone levels: right after exercising and when you're dehydrated.

Going forward, just monitor your ketones at a consistent time every time you do. If you test at 10:00 am today on Day 1, then always test at 10:00 am on future days. You're trying to find your baseline and your normal readings. Then, when it changes, you'll know!

Day 2

Today is your first attempt at Intermittent Fasting! We're going to do a skipped meal. Many Keto Dieters skip breakfast, because that's an easy meal to skip. A lot of us just aren't hungry in the mornings. Also, skipping breakfast extends your fast from the night before, increasing its benefits. You can skip lunch or skip dinner, too.

Whichever meal you decide to skip, make sure for the remainder of your meals, you're getting in your Macros. This means having extra Macro grams at the other meals than you normally would. How did this first day of fasting go? Were you hungry during the skipped meal period? Or, was it relatively easy? Record your experience.

Day 3

If Day 2 went well by both fasting and adding Macros to other meals, you're welcome to repeat it on Day 3. Pick a meal to skip and increase your Macros for the other meals.

If Day 2 was difficult and you were very hungry between meals, then just go back to a regular eating schedule on the Keto Diet. Cook and eat your three Ketogenic meals just like you normally would.

Day 4

Repeat Day 3. Skip one of your meals as your time spent Intermittent Fasting and eat your other meals with the increased Macro grams. Check to see that you're in ketosis using a monitoring tool. Track your Macros, your calories, and your Keto monitoring readout in a food diary.

Day 5

No Intermittent Fasting today. You are going to cook and eat your Keto meals as normal, with the Macros spread throughout the day. This gives your body a chance to rest between times of fasting. You may find as you proceed that you become more fat-adapted, which will slowly decrease your hunger. For those of you who like tracking data, you can check your ketones again today. Staying consistently in ketosis will help you lose the weight, too.

Day 6

Today, you'll practice Intermittent Fasting for a longer period. You're going to have an eating window of 10 hours, with 14 hours off for fasting. This eating window can start at any time in the morning and continue for the ten hours. For example, you could start it at 8:00 am and continue until 6:00 pm. After your eating window is done, you're not to eat any solid foods or broths until tomorrow. You can drink some water with lemon slices to keep up your electrolytes.

During your 10-hour eating window is when you'll consume all your Macros. You can split up the Macros into any meal combination you like. A heavy breakfast, light lunch, and heavy dinner would be an option. Or a combination that fits you. Don't forget to snack within those ten hours, so you can reach your Macro counts. Track everything in your food diary too.

Day 7

Yay, you've got to the end of your first week! Celebrate by weighing yourself. Have you lost any weight yet? A healthy weight loss schedule is up to two pounds per week. How are your energy levels? Are you doing well with the Intermittent Fasting times? Did you prefer the skipped meals or the 10-hour window? Tweak and adjust as the schedule go forward.

Today, you'll want to repeat Day 6 by doing another 10-hour window. It must be the exact same time as yesterday, to make sure you're getting the full fourteen-hour fasting cycle. So, if you started your ten-hour window at 8:00 am yesterday, you'll start it at 8:00 am today. Again, get all your Macros in your eating window. When it stops, that's when it's time to fast.

Week Two
Day 8

After several days of skipped meals and two days of 10-hour eating windows, it's time to shorten you're eating window and increase your fasting time. What time did your 10-hour eating window end yesterday? Count forward sixteen hours, and that's when your 8-hour eating window should start today. For example, if you ended your 10-hour window at 6:00 pm last night, you'll start your 8-hour eating window at 10:00 am today, and it will end at 6:00 pm. That's sixteen hours of fasting, consuming nothing but water with lemon slices for electrolytes. You'll want to eat all your Macros in your shorter 8-hour window. That includes breakfast, lunch, dinner, and your snack/dessert/drink.

Day 8 is also a good time to plan out meals for Week Two. Find recipes for those meals with the included Macros and go shopping for your ingredients to restock your kitchen. Also, monitor your ketones again. Are you staying in ketosis? If so, great! If not, adjust your Macros, follow the troubleshooting tips in the previous chapter, and get back into ketosis.

Day 9
The 8-hour feeding window from yesterday is repeated today, at the exact same time you started it yesterday. Eat all your Macros in the 8 hours. If you're having a bit of a challenge consuming enough of your Fat Macros in a shorter time frame, try taking some MCT oil. Start with a small amount, like a teaspoon, since it does cause nausea in some people. A 1 Tablespoon serving has 100 calories and 14 grams of good fats.

Day 10
Repeat your 16-hour Intermittent Fasting/8-hour Keto Dieting routine today as well. Just make sure you're consuming all your daily Macros in those 8 hours. If you're having difficulty, it's okay to go back to a regular Keto eating schedule. Adjust the eating window time, too, if it's not working out. If it is working out, great! After trying to fast for ten days, your body does start to change.

Day 11
Today is the day to not only continue your 16-hour fasting/8-hour eating plan, but to try incorporating some exercise into it. You don't have to, but getting exercise is wonderful for your body and has so

many benefits. You'll sleep better, too. Since your body is adjusting to a fasting schedule, don't overdo it on your workouts. A gentle 30-minute routine to get your heart rate up is usually all it takes. Just like yesterday, eat your Macros within the 8 hours. Track and record your experience.

Day 12

Today, we're going to shorten our eating window by one more hour, thus increasing our fasting window. You'll now be fasting for 17 hours and eating for 7 hours, and we'll repeat that cycle for several days. When was the end of yesterday's eating window? Count forward 17 hours, and that's when your 7-hour time frame begins. Now, you'll be eating all your Macros in a 7-hour period. Take your mineral supplements and gently increase your MCT oil dosage as well. Get plenty of water during fasting periods. You can add 30 minutes of exercise, but not if you are feeling weak or struggling with this eating routine. Give your body time to adjust.

Day 13

How did yesterday go when eating for just 7 hours during the day? The time goes by quick! By now, you should be able to tell when you're staying in ketosis even during those fasting times. It's noticeable! You'll feel it if you knock yourself out.

Repeat your 7-hour eating window schedule from yesterday. You can add exercise, too. Eat and track your Macros, making sure you're also getting your recommended calories. As eating windows get shorter, many Keto Dieters reduce the number of meals to two, plus a snack or Keto beverage. Eating twice a day works out for a lot of people, so give it a try!

Day 14

Congrats – you've reached the end of the second week. You went from a 10-hour window down to a 7-hour eating window, increasing your fasting time by three hours! That's three extra hours your body is spending pulling fuel sources from existing fat cells rather than relying on incoming fuel sources from your meals. You also added exercise, which burns even more fat in your cells. You've started to supercharge the Keto Diet effects by fasting.

It's time to assess the week. How did you do on your increased Intermittent Fasting? Was it easy to add exercise to it? Have you been tracking your Fats, Proteins, and Carbohydrates each day?

Weigh yourself to see if you've lost more weight. If so, excellent! If not, then you need to undertake some troubleshooting tips to help you. In addition to sticking to your 7-hour eating window today, check your ketones again using your monitor. Intermittent Fasting helps bump you into ketosis faster than simply cutting carbs. So, that's a noticeable change this week.

Week Three

Day 15

Day 15 begins with a new eating plan for this week, but now it's going to be based on a new eating window of just 6 hours. That's 18 hours spent fasting the rest of the time. Count forward from yesterday one additional hour, and that's when your fast should begin. You can adjust and tweak your fasting schedule during Days 15 and 16 to see which the best 6-hour timeframe for you is. But by Day 17, your routine should be consistent. Consistency with your feeding/fasting cycles is key to getting all the benefits from doing this.

You're also going to do your first 24-hour fast this week, so plan for that in your schedule. Go shopping for your Keto Diet ingredients and restock your cupboards. Make sure you have plenty of mineral rich foods for the day after your fast and keep a good supply of salty broths on hand, too.

Day 16

Today is the second day of your new 6-hour eating window and 18-hour fast. Eat all your Macros inside of those 6 hours and track them in your food diary. Are you feeling more energy? Many Keto Dieters enjoy such a short eating window, since it really makes the effects of fasting noticeable. You can add some exercise to your schedule as well. Start with 30 minutes and gradually increase, depending on your fitness goals and how well you're doing on your fasting/feeding cycles. It's okay to cut back on your fitness if you're feeling weak or sluggish in any way.

Day 17

Continue with your 6-hour feeding/18-hour fasting schedule today. Get in as many Macros as you can within those short six hours. Add your exercise to your routine, too. Make any adjustments like necessary. During fasting times, you should only be drinking water with a bit of lemon for electrolytes.

Day 18

Today is all about preparing for tomorrow's 24-hour fast. It's imperative that you eat all your Macros in their 6-hour feeding window today. Abstain from exercising, to give your muscles a chance to fully rest today and tomorrow. Check that you're in ketosis, too. If you're not, don't do the fast. Try a few more days of 18-hour fasts before you attempt a longer one. Once you're in ketosis, you can do a 24-hour fast.

Day 19

Today is your first 24-hour Intermittent Fasting day! Count 24 hours from the beginning of yesterday's fasting time and don't eat anything during that whole time. For example, if your 6-hour eating window ended at 6:00 pm yesterday, you're not to eat anything until 6:00 pm today.

Break your fast gently with some MCT oil and eat mineral rich foods like salmon, dark greens, avocado, nuts, and olives. Don't worry about getting in all your Macros but do stop all eating at least two hours before bedtime. Abstain from exercise today, too.

Day 20

Time to return to your 6-hour feeding/18-hour fasting cycle. How did yesterday's extended fast go? Make sure to rehydrate yourself today with plenty of water. Today, you do want to eat all your Macros just like you did on Day 18, even if you're not hungry. You're helping your body refuel itself with good fats. If you want to return to your exercise routine, you can if you feel up to it. Don't overdo it, though!

Day 21

Day 19's extended 24-hour fasting time was quite a challenge, but you got through it and did great! That's cause for celebration, and you can weigh yourself again, too. How close are you to meeting the weight loss goals you set before your monthly challenge began? If you've lost at least 5 pounds, then it's a good idea to go back to an online Macro calculator. Recalculate your Macros considering your new weight.

How is the 6-hour eating window going for you? If you prefer the 7-hour or the 8-hour timeframes, it's perfectly fine to return to those schedules instead! The important thing is to stay in ketosis. Check it again today using the Breath or Blood Monitor.

Week Four

Day 22

This week has an advanced 48-hour multi-day fasting time period that takes up Days 24 and Day 25. You're welcome to try it! Many of you have already experienced extraordinary health benefits just by doing the Intermittent Fasting so far, and we know you love a challenge! If at any point, you're feeling overwhelmed or sick or not enjoying the process in any way, it's okay to return to a normal Keto Diet schedule.

This is the beginning of the week, so it's a good idea to plan out your meals, shop for the ingredients, and stock your kitchen in preparation. Remember to purchase the mineral supplements and mineral-rich foods you'll need on Day 26 to break your fast. As for today, just continue your 6-hour eating window like you did yesterday.

Day 23

Today is about preparing for your multi-day fast, which begins tomorrow. Eat all your Macros within your 6-hour window, tracking them to make sure you've eaten enough good fats. Take note of the time your 6-hour window ends. You'll count 48 hours in advance, and that's when you can break your fast. Abstain from exercising today and throughout the fast as well. You can take light walks, but just don't be too strenuous on yourself.

Day 24

Fast all day today! Drink water take a mineral supplement and satisfy any hunger pangs with a small teaspoon of MCT oil. It's 100% good fats, and it won't affect either you are being in ketosis or take away the benefits of the fast.

Day 25

Fast all day today as well. Drink water take another mineral supplement, and you can have another teaspoon of MCT oil during the fast. Fast until it's been 48 hours since your Day 23 eating window ended. Break your fast with a low carb meal that includes mineral-rich foods like salmon, dark greens, and avocado. Don't try to get in your complete Macros before bedtime.

Day 26

Ease back into your 18-hour fast/6-hour eating window today. Eat your full Macros during those six hours. How did your 48-hour fast go? You can check your ketones to see how well you did! For most of you, staying in ketosis while fasting has really boosted its benefits!

Day 27

Repeat Day 26 with your normal 6-hour eating window. Today, though, you've given your body enough of a chance to rest from the effects of the 48-hour fast. So, you can add back in your regular exercise routine. Eat and track your Macros.

Day 28

Many congrats to you for getting through an amazing month of Keto Dieting and Intermittent Fasting! You can weigh yourself again and enjoy the results from your hard work. Go back to your food diary that you've been keeping throughout this month-long journey. Was it easier than you expected or more difficult? What was your personal experience with Intermittent Fasting? Casual 'fasters might want to stick with the skipped meals. More advanced 'fasters' really like the shorter eating windows. Those advanced 'fasters' looking to drop either their weight quickly or reach fitness goals quickly would do well to stay on shorter eating windows and incorporate longer fasts at least once a month.

However, your experience went, you deserve to celebrate! Show off your progress by posting "before" and "after" pictures of yourself.

Chapter 14:
Big No No's

Foods to Avoid: these foods are strictly out of bounds.

- All grains: wheat, oats, rye, quinoa, cereals, bread, millets, buckwheat, barley, corn

- Starchy vegetables: potatoes, yams, sweet potatoes

- Most fruits: bananas, apples, papayas, grapes, citrus, pears, peaches, pineapple, mangoes, nectarines

- Sugar: maple syrup, honey, basically anything with sugar

- Juice: all kinds as most juices come from sugary fruits

- Beans and legumes: this include all beans, chickpeas and lentils

- Alcohol: most alcoholic drinks have lots of sugar, so they are a big no-no (small amounts of dry wine in cooking is okay)

- Condiments and sauces: most bought sauces are high in sugars and carbs, so it's best to make your own out of simple, whole ingredients such as olive oil and vinegar.

Common Mistakes

With everything said and done, it should be mentioned that there are some common mistakes that are made by new Keto enthusiasts.

- Since no proper definition of how much carb is actually "Low-Carb" exists, some people often tend to shoot their carb intake to a very high level while still considering that they are under "Low-Carb." The level of daily carb should be around 20-50 for an optimal experience, but a maximum of 100-150g.

- It is understood that as a macronutrient, protein is very important as a bodybuilding food. It improves the level of satiety and encourages fat burning. Yet, be aware of having too much protein as the excess might turn into glucose, which will once more be burned up for energy instead of fat.

- A very big mistake made by newcomers is they naturally think that lowering the level of fat alongside the carbs might increase the fat loss. That is wrong! Keep in mind that you need the fat in your body if you want to encourage the burning of fat!

- When on Keto, you need to reduce the level of insulin. While on a Ketogenic diet, your insulin levels will go down significantly, which helps greatly to relieve the level of bloat. Still, with that very process, electrolytes from our body are also flushed away. Therefore, balance the decrease in electrolytes by having a good amount of sodium (salt) intake to make sure that your kidneys are safe, and you don't have problems such as fatigue, constipation or a light headache.

Mistake #1: Hidden Carbs

Not counting hidden carbohydrates is one of the most common mistakes committed while on Ketogenic diet. First, food manufacturers are not completely accurate with the amount of carbohydrates on their labels. Read ingredients on the packaged food and make sure there are not any ingredients on there that would account for some extra carbohydrates. Those hidden carbs can add up fast.

The second way this can happen is when you look at the ingredients and see that there are carbohydrates, but you fail to look at the serving size. For example, some candies and candy bars are listed as two servings, meaning you need to double the amount of carbohydrates on the package if you plan on eating the entire thing!

Mistake #2: Sweeteners and Fruit

Fruit contains a ton of excess carbohydrates in the form of fructose, especially when it's completely ripened. Limit your fruit consumption or you will go over your carb limit very quickly.

Mistake #3: Too Much Protein

In excess, protein can convert into glucose via gluconeogenesis. You want to burn ketones, not glucose. Ketogenic diet, protein makes up approximately 25% of your calories.

Mistake #4: Not Eating Enough!

If you are not eating enough, and severely restrict your calories, you will feel hungry. You will likely get irritable, and the diet won't last. For lasting results, stick to the 70% fats, 25% protein, 5% carbs. You'll be eating a lot fatter than on a normal diet, this might take some adjustment.

Mistake #5: Not Enough Sodium

Get salty. During ketosis, insulin levels reduce greatly. Lowered insulin triggers the kidneys to dump sodium. Increase sodium intake to avoid deficiency. Sea salt is healthiest.

The only thing left now is to know what you need and going to do, to prepare yourself for the journey ahead.

Chapter 15:
Tips and Tricks and FAQs

There are important considerations you need to know before you embark on the Ketogenic diet. Below are some important tips to recap and help you be successful with this diet.

Tip #1: Count Carbohydrates

There are some useful apps out there you can find on your phone or online calculators to count net carbohydrates. However, there is a simple way to do this. When in doubt, simply take the total carbohydrates listed on a product's label and subtract the fiber from that total amount. This is your net carbohydrates. Of course, if you're eating fresh, whole foods, this is a little more difficult because there isn't any label packaging. That's where apps are handy.

Tip #2: Planning and Preparation

Planning for this diet, you need to shop for the right foods and cook at home more. Creating and following a meal plan is key to success. Sit down and outline your day/week/month, and don't forget to plan for snacks!

Tip #3: Eat Enough Fat
With this diet, fat makes up 70% of your caloric intake. That's a lot of fat. In order to get enough calories, stock up on the fat. Even if you are in a calorie deficit, you're still eating 70% fat. If you're having trouble getting enough fat, stock up on the olive oil, coconut oil and butter. You'll be eating a lot of these fats, bulk purchase to save money.

Tip #4: Make Keto A Lifestyle
It's a good idea to try turning the Ketogenic diet into a lifestyle plan. This means making the diet into a habit. In order to do this, you should first try not to overwhelm yourself and don't get upset if you backpedal and don't follow the plan. Immediately return to it and try again.

Commitment is key! Commit to the Ketogenic diet for a week, two weeks, and then maybe a month. By the end of a month, it will turn into a habit and living this new lifestyle won't seem as difficult.

Tip #5: Drink Plenty of Water
Entering a stage of ketosis will naturally deplete your body's water supply. Therefore, you need to drink tons of water in order to stay hydrated, but not only that, you need to keep an eye on your electrolyte levels too.

Tip #6: Increase Salt Intake

As levels of insulin circulating through your body lower, your kidneys will begin excreting some excess sodium. Eat more salt to avoid electrolyte deficiency.

Tip #7: Experiment
Have fun with this diet! Although there are restrictions, compared to most diets, it's flexible and so delicious. Play around with recipes and different ingredients. Enjoy trying new foods you might have never explored, just make sure you're following your macros.

Tip #8: Keto + Intermittent Fasting
A common practice for rapid weight loss is combining Ketogenic diet with intermittent fasting. This is common as many people find it easier and more convenient to meet their macros with this pattern of eating. Intermittent fasting is a pattern of eating in which you cycle between periods of fasting (fasted state) and eating (fed state).

Tip #9: Patience
Be patient. Follow the diet, and the results will show over time. Don't stress out if results don't show up immediately. Good things come to those who are disciplined and have patience. Eating more carbs will be tempting, if you really want the results, stick to your macros.

- Cook for yourself – freeze the remaining servings or save half of the recipes, if needed.

- Swap your meals – you can swap your meals any time of the day. Eat breakfast for lunch or lunch for dinner. Your meal plan depends on you!

- Try to skip the snacks – while you should feel satisfied with the 3 main meals, keep Keto-friendly snacks close by.

- Only eat when hungry – if you don't feel hunger, don't eat.

- Substitute – fish, pork, and lamb can be substituted for one another in recipes due to their similar nutritional value.

Understand that diet plans are not suitable for everyone: Make sure that your daily requirements match your recipes and diet plan. Make small adjustments and reduce the portions if needed. Don't worry if you go over your protein intake a bit, as it will not kick you out of ketosis and will keep hunger at bay. If you find yourself lacking enough fat in your diet, add more fat by adding oils and fatty foods according to your adjustments.

Tips for Going Out

The Ketogenic diet can seem easy enough for the times when you are cooking your own food at home, but it can be quite a challenge to eat out at dining establishments or social events if you are not prepared. When going to a restaurant, call ahead or look at the menu before you arrive and see what they have. Keep an eye out for grilled or steamed vegetables and see if they can poach an egg if you need some extra protein. Otherwise, have a snack before you go out and simply order a vegetable side. If you can find a restaurant that serves breakfast items all day, you are all set! Just be sure to stay away from industrial oils like canola, and always ask they your food be prepared with pure olive oil or butter.

Often the salad dressings served in restaurants are loaded with unhealthy oils and sugar. If you believe that you may be enjoying a side of vegetables or a salad as your entrée, ask if they can provide you with a lemon and some pure extra virgin olive oil to use as a dressing along with some salt and black pepper. Otherwise, you could sneak in a small bottle of extra virgin olive oil just in case they do not have any of their own to serve. Keep in mind that many restaurants serve what they call an "olive oil blend," which is olive oil blended with canola oil. Most of the time, you can pretty much bet that what they are giving you is not pure unless you specifically ask, or even state that you have a severe allergy. This makes them more likely to take your request seriously.

When going to a social event, the best course of action is almost always to bring a dish. Choose something that is substantial enough to be eaten on its own, like a salad with plenty of nuts. If you happen to be in a dinner party where everything is to be prepared for you and you do not have the option to bring a dish of your own, have a chat with the host and explain to him or her that you have special dietary needs. If he or she will be cooking meat as the main dish, find out what sides are being prepared. If any of them are low in carbohydrates, perhaps imply that they could make an additional amount of that side so that you may enjoy it as your main course. You can always have a quick snack before you arrive, such as a hard-boiled egg or some nuts for protein and fat.

Tips for Staying Optimum Ketosis Level

1) Testing Ketone Levels – the most inexpensive way to do this is testing your urine for acetoacetate, the ketone measured in urine. The test can be carried out early in the morning or after dinner when on a Keto diet. You will just dip the ketone urine strips in your urine. The darker the strip the higher the ketone levels are and the better that it is. The shades can range from pink to purple.

2) Sustained and Ample Protein Consumption – the keyword here is ample which does not equate to excessive protein intake. The suggested formula to use is multiplying your body weight in pounds by 0.55 to 0.77; for example, your ideal weight is 140-lbs then your protein intake daily should be between 77g to 107.8g.

3) Go into a Fat Fast or Short Fast – this is going for fasts like an intermittent fasting. Example of a short fast is to go fasting for at least 14 hours in between dinner and your breakfast the next day to induce ketosis. Fat fasting on the other hand is just eating 1,000 calories in one day with the bulk of the food coming from fats. You can do this once or twice a week to induce ketosis.

4) Boost Your Intake of healthy Fats – since the Keto diet is composed mostly between 80%-90% fats, it is only sensible to consume the healthy types of fats and they are coconut oil, butter, avocado oil, olive oil, and the likes. And if you are on a Keto diet to lose weight, mind your calories too.

5) Increase your Physical Activity – studies show that when you are physically active, it increases your ketone levels. But, if you're still new to the Keto diet, it may take your body one to four weeks to adapt to this new metabolic pathway and hence physical performance can be temporarily reduced.

6) Add Coconut Oil in the Diet – coconut oil is a type of fat known as medium-chain triglycerides (MCTs) and studies have shown that this type of fat can create a more sustained level of ketosis.

7) Strictly Lower Carb Intake – Remember the first pathway that the body uses? By breaking down carbs into glucose and then using glucose as fuel for the bodily processes? That's what you completely need to avoid in order to get into a ketosis. It is suggested that if you want to lose weight fewer than 21 grams of carb consumption daily is the paramount goal.

Tips for Working Out While on Keto and IF
It's okay to exercise on an empty stomach: Many people believe exercising on an empty stomach reduces performance. They also

believe exercising on an empty stomach will cause muscle loss and not the desired fat loss.

This is not true! You still have fat as an energy source. The only time your body starts to digest the proteins for fuel is when you aren't getting enough fat in your diet.

Another point worth mentioning is the type of exercise and diet. Muscle loss can occur with certain types of exercise, not based on whether you eat before exercising. Calorie restrictive diets or eating too little can contribute to muscle loss. You lose muscle not because you fasted before exercising but rather because you are generally not eating enough.

Too much cardio can also be a culprit in muscle loss. Many health and fitness experts recommend weightlifting over cardio to lose weight. This also helps tone the body while burning fats.

Exercises to perform while fasting or on ketogenesis: Some conditions promote muscle loss while excess fat is minimally burned. One is when you lose a lot of weight too fast within a short period. Another is when you eat too little but exercise a lot. Another is simply exercising too much with the wrong type of workout.

The intensity of the exercise is important when exercising in a Ketogenic state. You must aim to train with low intensity until your body is well adapted to the diet. High-intensity exercises for a long period require glucose, which you do not have in abundance during ketogenesis. Your body cannot produce ketones quickly enough to supply you with energy for long intense workouts. If you train during fasting periods, use low-intensity exercises. Steady-state, lower intensity cardio aerobic or cardio exercises work well.

Anaerobic exercise such as HIIT or weightlifting should be avoided until you are adapted and should not be done on fasting days. If you need, or want, to train with higher intensity during ketogenesis and find that your performance is limited by Keto, follow a targeted Keto diet. Eat fast-acting carbohydrate foods 30 minutes before a workout. One example is fruit. Limit the number of carbohydrates to 15 to 30 grams only. That will be enough to fuel your HIIT, especially if you do long HIIT workouts. I stick to 20-minute HIIT workouts and never need to add in carbs. Listen to your body and adjust as needed.

More Favorite Tips and Tricks

Plan Your Meals Smartly: Start your meal planning in advance and determine which foods you will need to prepare the meals for the whole week. Use your free time to prepare these foods in advance and store in refrigerator/freezer in containers. Similarly, make a list of food to purchase, go to grocery store and purchase ingredients for the whole week and store in your fridge and pantry.

Pick the Right Containers: Purchase containers according to your freezer size and your requirements. Always purchase containers that are BPA free and freezer safe. Similarly, buy bowls that are oven and microwave safe, so that you can re-heat the recipes in your bowl and serve them warm.

Use Frozen Vegetables: When it comes to preparing vegetables and fruits such as tomatoes, avocado, onions, cucumber, etc. Just chop them or make them as per recipe direction and store them in containers in the freezer. Frozen prepared vegetables save a lot of your time to prepare recipes as all you need to do is just to take them out from the freezer, thaw them and use directly to make recipes.

Store in Advance: For smoothies, you can place all the ingredients in fridge or freezer and blend them whenever you want to make smoothies. Similarly, you can prepare all your desserts in advance and store in the freezer. You can have them whenever you want. You can also prepare them in more quantity so that you can use them to serve on multiple days.

Be Patient to Master the Skill: Always remember that prepping meals requires some time to learn perfectly and will get better with experience. So, if you end up spoiling some ingredients, it's very normal. Try with simple recipes and try storing a few components first and then move up the ladder. Don't rush into learning everything at once.

Frequently Asked Questions

By now, you are aware of what is meant by Keto diet and intermittent fasting, and what you might expect from choosing to implement as your lifestyle. Here are some frequently asked questions to cover all relevant information. You can also use this section as a quick reference guide.

Q: How long will it take to get into ketosis?

The Ketogenic diet is not one that you can use intermittently, as you might with a fad diet. Its intention is not being a quick fix. As with any change that impacts our body, it takes a while to adjust and eventually reach the state of ketosis. It can take from 2 days to a whole week, give or take a little, considering your body, how much physical activity you are doing, and what you are (or aren't) eating. Some say that the fastest means of achieving ketosis is to do physical activity as much as possible on an empty stomach (like intermittent fasting), restricting your carb intake to no more than 20 grams a day, and maintaining proper hydration and electrolytes.

Q: Do I have to count calories?

Calories are going to matter at the end of the day. For weight loss, you need a calorie deficit and counting calories can be useful. However, it is time-consuming and tedious. Your job is to eat properly and never go too far into a deficit or too far over your limit. With the Ketogenic diet, you don't have to worry about calories as much because the fats and proteins fill you up and keep you feeling full for a longer period. However, if you exercise, you might want to be vigilant.

Q: Is it possible to eat too much fat?

Yes, it is possible to eat too much fat. In the end, you must be calorie deficit in order to lose weight. While most people are going to find it hard to overeat on a low carbohydrate high-fat diet, it is still possible to do. Calculate your macros and stick with those in order to lose weight. If your objective is maintaining your weight, or gain weight, you can eat even more fat.

Q: How much weight will I lose?

As with achieving ketosis, this is very individual. It depends not only on what you're eating (slightly more or fewer carbs or fat) and how much exercise you're getting but also just your genetic makeup. If you add a lot of exercise to your regimen, you will speed up and sometimes even increase your total amount of weight loss. You can also eliminate certain foods that may cause your weight loss to slow, like artificial sweeteners like Splenda (science suggests these actually can cause weight gain), wheat products or wheat-contaminated products (anything that may have trace amounts, especially if you might have an intolerance), dairy products, and low-fat processed foods. In the initial days or weeks, you may notice a very rapid weight loss. Unfortunately, this isn't fat, but rather, water loss. The Keto diet is a diuretic, which means you'll be having to urinate a lot more frequently, and it'll seem like you've lost a lot of weight, even though it's just water. On the upside, this means that your body is adjusting and likely heading towards ketosis, which is exactly what you want. It's in this state of ketosis that you'll really start burning off some fat.

Q: I started this diet, and now I don't feel good. What's going on?

As your body adjusts to this new state, it's very common for you to feel a bit under the weather and flu-like. Many people report experiencing headaches and some brain fogginess as well. Like mentioned before, ketosis causes a diuretic state, which means losing a lot of water from your body. With the drastic water loss and the consumption of our last remaining stores of glycogen, you're peeing out important electrolytes and you need to replace them ASAP. You need to be always hydrated by ensuring that you drink lots of water, and make sure to bump up your salt intake as well. Jerky, bacon, sausage, pepperoni, salted nuts, and even broths (both meat and veggie) are all excellent choices for getting the sodium you need. Replacing your electrolytes and staying properly hydrated will help lessen the "Keto flu" while your body adjusts. Remember to stay on top of these things even after being on the diet for a significant amount of time, as a drop-in electrolyte at any time will cause you to feel pretty icky.

Q: I have stopped losing weight, what's gone wrong and what can I do?

With any kind of new diet and exercise routine, weight loss plateaus happen, and the Ketogenic diet is no exception. There are various things that can cause this problem, but luckily there are also several things that you can try to help you get around this rut. You can try intermittent fasting, changing your workout routine, tweaking your diet - or all these things if you're really looking to shatter the plateaus. Try out the following in the given to change things up and begin burning off more fat:

- Cut out dairy products entirely, both low-fat and full fat
- Increase fat intake of healthy varieties
- Drop your carbohydrate daily intake even further
- Stop eating certain kinds of nuts and seeds (like cashews, which are highest in fat) or all kinds entirely
- Cut out gluten-containing products altogether, as well as gluten-contaminated (processes with gluten-containing foods even though it might not contain it itself) if you are sensitive to gluten
- Cut out sweeteners, including honey, syrups, and artificial sweeteners
- Track all your carbs and calories (macros in general) so you can make sure nothing is sneaking in
- Cut out processed foods

Progress isn't always about decreasing the number on the scale; for this reason, considering switching to measuring (chest, waist, thighs, upper arms) instead of weighing. This way you get a more accurate account of your progress.

Q: Should I take any supplement while on the Keto diet?

It's always a good idea to talk to a qualified medical professional on this subject, but because it's pretty common for people to get muscle cramps or just feel a bit off after starting a Ketogenic diet, there are some supplements that have been recommended to help with those issues. These supplements include:

- Multivitamins for your specific gender, condition, lifestyle, and age
- Mineral supplement that contains potassium, magnesium, and other trace minerals to support your electrolyte balance
- Vitamin B (full spectrum) Complex
- Vitamin D with Calcium Supplement

Consult your medical practitioner or nutritionist to address your individual needs.

Q: Is eating all this fat bad for me? What about heart attacks?

There are three known primary fat categories: saturated fats, polyunsaturated fats, and monounsaturated fats. In the past, we thought that saturated fats were responsible for a lot of rising health issues, and there seemed to be a lot that connected these fats to a plethora of health problems, specifically heart disease. In recent years, however, science has discovered that saturated fats are not to blame for heart attacks but can also help to improve cholesterol levels. Polyunsaturated fats, however, are a bit trickier to understand. Polyunsaturated fats are commonly found in processed foods and condiments, particularly those with hydrogenated vegetable oils, are notably unhealthy for a number of reasons, plus they usually have a lot of trans fats; trans fats have legitimately been connected to heart disease and other health issues (like obesity) and therefore should be avoided.

On the other hand, there are also polyunsaturated fats that occur naturally in certain foods, like fish and certain kinds of eggs, which are quite beneficial for us; these good fats have shown to help balance cholesterol levels, for example. So be sure to include sources of these healthy, naturally found kinds of fats, and try your best to eliminate the unnatural, unhealthy varieties. Lastly, we have monounsaturated fats. These are typically healthy and can be eaten without worry. Olive oil, for example, is more proportionately a monounsaturated fat, which is healthy for us and can help with lowering our cholesterol.

Q: Isn't fasting only a "fad" and can it really help me lose weight?

Fasting is not a fad as it has been utilized for thousands of years in medicine, various cultures and religions. It wasn't invented yesterday. In addition, fasting can help you lose weight and maintain it. The key is to find the fasting protocol that works best for you in conjunction with a low carbohydrate high-fat eating program to achieve the benefits you desire.

Q: Isn't fasting just another name for "starvation"?

While many may think so, fasting is not starvation. Fasting can be defined as a voluntary act of not eating for a specific time period.

Q: Won't you always be hungry with fasting? Will it cause you to overeat?

This is one of most asked questions as we have all experienced various weight loss programs where we are constantly hungry. First and foremost, if you eliminate processed foods and primarily eat whole foods (primarily transition to a low carbohydrate high-fat diet), the lowering of empty carbohydrates will help reduce your constant hunger pangs.

Because refined and highly processed foods have much of their fiber, essential nutrients, minerals and fats removed with sugar and other processed ingredients added back in, these types of carbohydrates enter quickly into your bloodstream where no satiety mechanisms are triggered to tell you that you are full. While this is occurring, your insulin levels skyrocket. When your insulin rises to a very high level, it indicates your body to store fat, but you are still hungry, so you eat more and store more fat. Thus, you are in a never-ending cycle of storing fat and continue to gain weight.

Such foods like fresh leafy green vegetables contain many nutrients and important fiber that triggers the satiety receptors as your stomach stretches. Both protein and fats trigger satiety mechanisms which also indicate when you are full to stop eating.

Q: I have never fasted before. Is it safe and is it hard to do?

As I previously mentioned, fasting has been around for thousands of years and one of the most used therapies in medicine. Fasting is not a new fad or something that appeared from nowhere. Therefore, it is safe if you first consult with your medical doctor and receive concurrence.

Believe it or not, you are fasting every night during your sleep. While it may be about 6 to 8 hours per night depending on your sleep patterns, your body is working to repair and rejuvenate itself for the next day.

Q: Don't you lose electrolytes with fasting?

There exist several discussions on loss of electrolytes and malnutrition during fasting, but the main issue is really about the deficiency of micronutrients. Studies have not found any evidence of malnutrition during prolonged fasts. Some of the key points are:

- Potassium levels only decreased slightly and without the use of any supplements

- Calcium, phosphorous and magnesium levels were stable as just about all the calcium and phosphorous are stored in our bones.

Q: Can you exercise when you are fasting?

Many believe that you should not exercise when fasting. There is no reason why you should not exercise unless you have some medical or physical condition preventing you. However, I suggest you start exercising once you transition to a fasting regimen for a couple of weeks, so your body becomes adapted to fasting. Start slow and progress with your exercise program over time. Don't be in a hurry. You are beginning a new healthy lifestyle change so don't overstress your body all at once. Exercise can be safely done with fasting but preferably during a fasted state for the best results.

Q: Can anyone fast?

Fasting can be done by many but there are exceptions. Children, the sick and elderly, underweight adults, pregnant and women breastfeeding, and those with serious medical conditions should not attempt fasting. Those who are on medications and have health issues must always speak to their doctor first before attempting to fast or start any new diet or physical exercise program.

Conclusion

Now that you have finished this book, it is only natural to be extremely anxious to get started not only with the Keto diet but with intermittent fasting as well. Nevertheless, it is important to follow the steps outlined in the chapters and start with the Keto diet before adding in intermittent fasting after your body has had the time it needs to adjust to the change, which should be a minimum of one month.

While you may be anxious to get started losing as much weight as possible, forcing your body to adapt to both lifestyle changes at once is likely to cause it to feel as though you are in a situation where it needs to hold on to every single calorie possible, curtailing weight loss in the process. Instead, it is important to give your body the time it needs to adjust and realize that following the Ketogenic diet while fasting intermittently is more akin to a marathon than a sprint which means that slow and steady wins the race.

Adhere to the outlined steps and make the journey a success. Good luck!

Christine Moore

If you find this book helpful in anyway a review to support my endeavors is much appreciated.

www.ingramcontent.com/pod-product-compliance
Lightning Source LLC
Chambersburg PA
CBHW020257030426
42336CB00010B/810